The Homecare Workers' H

C000193043

Published by:
United Kingdom Homecare Association Limited (UKHCA)
Group House
52 Sutton Court Road
Sutton
Surrey SM1 4SL

Registered in England No. 3083104

ISBN 978-0-9534243-7-5

Contents

Introduction

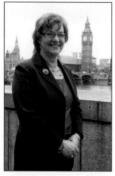

Bridget Warr
Chief Executive, UKHCA

Giving someone the opportunity and ability to continue to live at home and in their community is one of the most important jobs in society today.

With the number of people who need support to live independently at home set to grow rapidly this century, as the older population grows larger and medical advances mean more children with disabilities achieve adulthood, your role will become even more crucial.

It's essential there is a knowledgeable workforce with the expertise to carry out day to day care tasks, from helping people get up, wash and dress and take their medication, to the complex support required by someone who needs oxygen or whose dementia leaves them without the ability to make sense of the world.

As someone who sees service users daily, or almost daily, your contribution, as a careworker, to their well-being is vital. Homecare is not as simple as making someone a cup of tea, though this sort of support and companionship is essential for people's well-being. Careworkers also need to know how to monitor changes in their service users' health and demeanour, what to do in an emergency and how best to support family carers who may be stretched by the demands of caring.

The UKHCA Homecare Workers' Handbook is designed to be a portable guide for new careworkers or more experienced staff who would like to refresh their knowledge.

It is intended to supplement, not replace employers' policies and procedures, and has been written as a general guide to homecare across the UK. This new handbook replaces the second edition of our previous handbook, published in 2003.

Thank you for your commitment to this important area of work. We hope you will enjoy your work and value being a member of the huge band of caring, sensitive and knowledgeable people who make homecare in the UK a service to be proud of.

Bridget Warr

Chief Executive, UKHCA

About this handbook

Who is it for?

This handbook is for careworkers – in particular those who work for organisations that are members of United Kingdom Homecare Association (UKHCA).

This handbook is written for those of you who are employed by a homecare provider. However, if you are self-employed or employed by your service user, most of the guidance in this handbook will still apply to you, even though the relationship between you, your agency and the service user will be different.

How should you use it?

The handbook is designed to be portable, so that you can carry it with you and refer to it whenever you need guidance on a particular topic.

You may decide to read through the handbook as part of your induction if you are new to care work, or to refresh your knowledge if you are experienced in the role. The handbook can also be used as the basis for discussions with your supervisor or with colleagues as part of your professional development, or simply used for reference.

Remember that you should read and follow your employer's policies, procedures and guidance. Where these are different from the guidance in this handbook, follow your employer's policies, as there may be tasks or actions described in this handbook that are outside your role description or not permitted under your employer's policies.

Describing roles and organisations

In this handbook we use the following words to describe the organisations and people that play a part in homecare:

- Careworker – sometimes known as a domiciliary careworker, support worker, personal carer or caregiver.

- Employer/Agency/Organisation – the homecare organisation that you work for.

- Service user – someone who receives support from a careworker.

- Supervisor – the person who manages you, or who is your first point of contact at the organisation you work for. You may also know them as a line manager, manager, coordinator or team leader.

- Family carer – a family member or friend who looks after a service user without being paid.

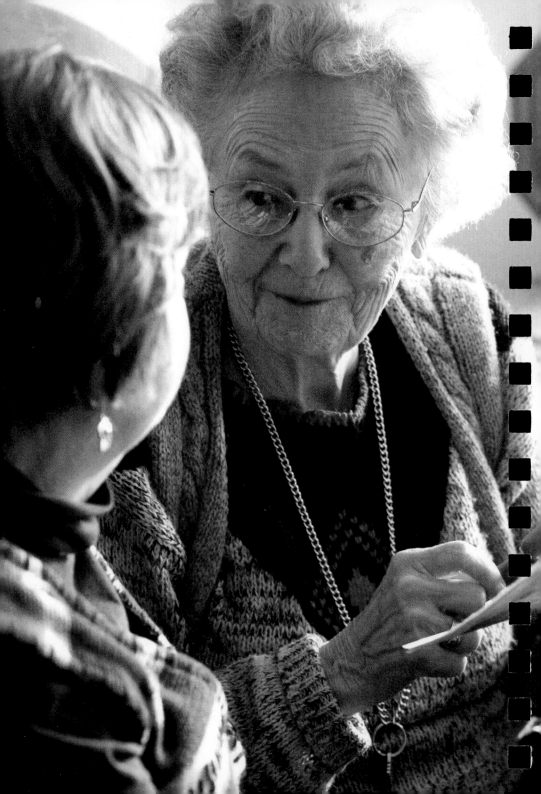

1   Principles of good care practice

The care and support you provide will be informed by a set of good practice principles. These are the values that act as the foundation for the delivery of good care.

Regulatory bodies, professional associations and individual homecare agencies have their own codes of practice, values or principles. If you are working towards a vocational qualification, your course will be based on a framework of good practice principles.

Think about how you can apply these principles to your day-to-day work – both in terms of the way you carry out practical tasks and how you interact with service users. If there's anything you don't understand, discuss it with your supervisor or during training.

While they may be written in slightly different ways, most organisations' good practice principles are likely to include the following:

- Personal choice – service users have the right to make decisions about their lives.

- Rights – service users' rights should always be respected. These include their human rights and legal rights.

- Independence – service users should be supported to live as independently as possible. This means enabling them to do as much as they can for themselves.

- Respect and dignity – service users should always be treated with respect and dignity.

- Individuality – every person is unique, and service users will all have different backgrounds, characters, abilities and skills. The individuality of each service user must be recognised.

- Freedom from discrimination – service users should not be disadvantaged in their treatment because of their: age, race, disability or gender; or because of their religion or beliefs; or because they are pregnant or on maternity leave; or because of their marital or civil partnership status, their sexual orientation or because of gender re-assignment.

- Privacy and confidentiality – service users have the right for information about them to remain confidential and to have their privacy respected.

- Compliments and complaints – service users have the right to comment on the care services they receive and to have complaints dealt with in an open and effective way.

- Freedom from abuse – service users have the right to remain safe and free from abuse and neglect by anyone, including: careworkers, health workers, family members, friends, representatives or any other carers.

2 Standards and regulations in the homecare sector

This chapter explains the broader context in which standards for the provision of homecare are set and enforced.

Professional standards

United Kingdom Homecare Association (UKHCA) is the professional association of homecare providers from the independent, voluntary, not-for-profit and statutory sectors.

If your employer or agency is a UKHCA member, it must comply with the UKHCA Code of Practice.

The Code sets out the rights of service users in relation to the care they receive and the agency's responsibilities to careworkers. It also outlines the standards that relate to the running of the agency and its legal and financial responsibilities.

Your employer can give you a copy of the UKHCA Code of Practice, or it is available at: www.ukhca.co.uk/codeofpractice.aspx

Regulation of careworkers

Careworkers may also be subject to registration with a workforce regulator. Registered careworkers are required to abide by a professional code of practice and may be required to demonstrate their fitness to practice annually and in the event of a misconduct hearing.

Your employer will tell you whether or not you need to be registered in the part of the UK in which you work.

At the time of writing the workforce regulators are:

- In Northern Ireland – the Northern Ireland Social Care Council. www.niscc.info/

- In Scotland – the Scottish Social Services Council. www.sssc.uk.com/

- In Wales – the Care Council for Wales. www.ccwales.org.uk/

- In England – The workforce regulator has not been confirmed at the time of writing.

Regulation of homecare providers

There are several statutory organisations which play a part in setting standards for homecare in the UK and making sure homecare providers meet those standards. They are known as regulators or regulatory bodies. Each has its own standards for the delivery of care, and the agency you work for will be monitored and inspected by its regulator. You may be asked to speak to an inspector at some point in your work. You should answer their questions honestly.

Homecare in the UK is regulated by the following bodies:

- in England – the Care Quality Commission (CQC). www.cqc.org.uk/

- in Wales – Care and Social Services Inspectorate Wales (CSSIW). www.wales.gov.uk/cssiwsubsite/newcssiw/

- in Scotland – the Care Inspectorate. www.scswis.com/

- in Northern Ireland – the Regulation and Quality Improvement Authority (RQIA). www.rqia.org.uk/

Your agency will usually be required to register with the relevant regulator in order to provide homecare.

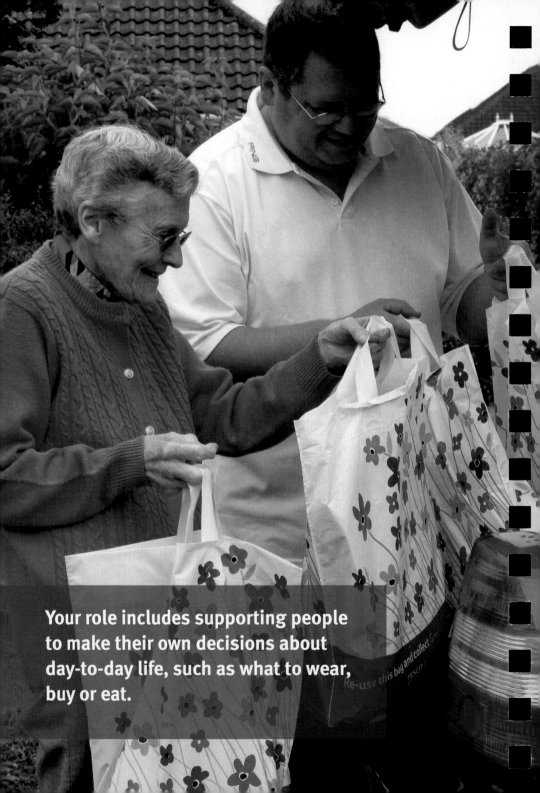

Your role includes supporting people to make their own decisions about day-to-day life, such as what to wear, buy or eat.

3   Your role

As a careworker, you do one of the most important jobs in the community today. In everything you do, you'll need to think about the care and support you provide from the service user's point of view, so that their rights and choices are always respected. By helping service users to carry out everyday tasks you make a big difference to their lives. As a careworker you are:

- Supporting people to live independently at home, so they can continue to live in the way they wish. This helps to maintain their individuality, independence and self-esteem.

- Enabling people to stay in familiar surroundings, to take part in their usual activities and to be part of their community.

- Helping to maintain their health and wellbeing through the support you offer, and by recognising when people need specialist help or treatment from another professional.

- Supporting people to make their own decisions about day-to-day life, such as what to wear, buy or eat.

- Providing social contact. A friendly face and a chat can be important for everyone, especially those who live on their own.

- Helping other carers – such as service users' family members, to continue to care for their loved one.

Your work will be very rewarding, but it is complex and can sometimes be challenging. As well as common sense, kindness and good humour, you will need to develop a range of professional skills, knowledge and personal attributes. For example, you will:

- Support people from different backgrounds, cultures and lifestyles, so you will need to be open-minded, sensitive and non-judgemental. Your own beliefs or opinions must not affect the service you provide or the way you treat service users.

- Support people with many different health issues, so you will need to understand different conditions and how they affect people. You will also need to be able to spot any signs of ill-health or changes in a person's wellbeing and help them to get the necessary treatment or care by reporting concerns to your supervisor.

- Help people to do as much as possible for themselves rather than doing things for them, so you'll need patience and understanding in order to avoid the temptation to 'take over'.

- Help people to carry out intimate or personal tasks, so you'll need tact, sensitivity and the ability to build a good relationship with people so that they feel comfortable with you. You also need to know the steps you can take to help maintain their privacy and dignity to avoid people feeling embarrassed.

- Need to be conscientious and dependable, so you must arrive as punctually as you can, and carry out tasks to the best of your ability.

- Be faced with the unexpected, so you'll need to know what to do in an emergency.

You and your employer

Your employer has certain responsibilities towards you as an employee, such as ensuring your working environment is safe and that you have the support you need to do your job. As an employee you also have responsibilities towards your employer. These include:

- Keeping your side of the agreement or contract you make with your employer, and following the policies and procedures that apply to your work.

- Keeping yourself informed and updated about all aspects of care practice. You must stay up to date and develop your knowledge, skills and understanding by undertaking training, whether or not it is provided by your employer.

- Being prepared for emergencies. See *Chapter 7 – What to do in an emergency* and read it from time to time so that you know what to do in an emergency situation. It is important to understand the procedures to follow if an accident or sudden illness occurs while you are at work, but you should also be aware of emergency first aid procedures that you are **not** allowed to carry out at your level of training.

- Telling your employer if you are concerned about your health or your work, or if you, or somebody else may feel unsafe. See *Chapter 5 – Health and safety at work*.

- Your employer will need to be able to demonstrate that all relevant insurance cover is in place. You should, therefore, provide them with up to date documentation for their records.

While at work, you are accountable for your actions. As well as supporting you, part of your supervisor's role is to make sure you are doing your job properly, so that service users receive the best possible care and are not put at risk.

It is important that you keep your supervisor up-to-date with any concerns or problems you come across at work, so that you and your service users, get the support that you need.

Resolving problems at work

Your employer should give you a copy of their grievance procedure. This is the formal process that can be used by staff to raise a complaint with their employer. Usually the grievance procedure would only be used as a last resort where it has not been possible to resolve the problem informally, for example by talking about it during supervision.

Taking care of yourself

To provide a high standard of support to other people, you need to take good care of yourself, both physically and emotionally.

Care work is physically demanding and it's important that you try to eat well and get enough sleep, so you have the energy necessary in order to provide good care.

Always follow your employer's directions about health and safety and your training. For example, only helping a service user to move using the techniques and equipment you have learned about in training.

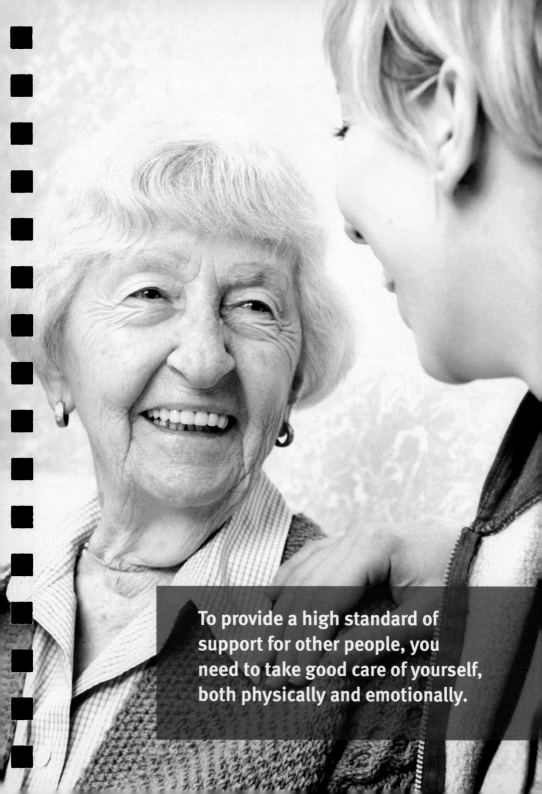

To provide a high standard of support for other people, you need to take good care of yourself, both physically and emotionally.

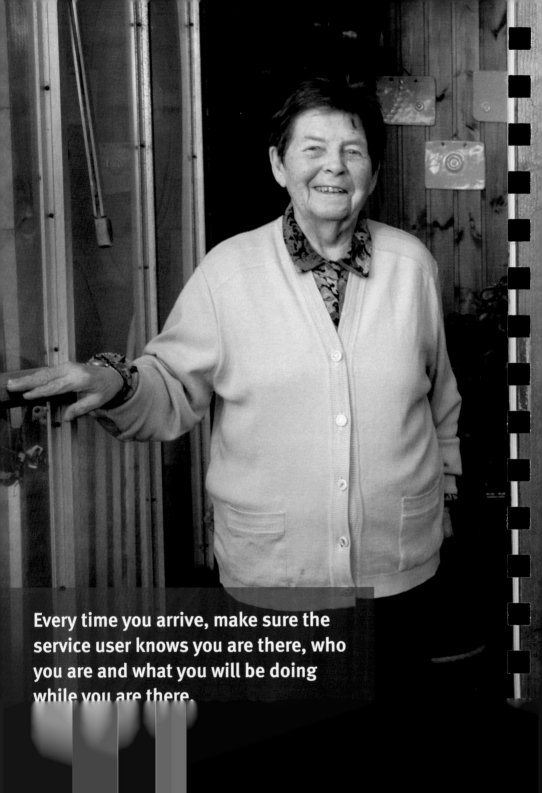

Every time you arrive, make sure the service user knows you are there, who you are and what you will be doing while you are there.

4   Service users and their homes

During the course of your work you will meet a wide variety of service users. They will all have different personalities and different support needs. The service users you work with could be young or old, or may have dementia, learning disabilities or mental health needs.

You will need to use your skills and knowledge across a broad range of situations and treat each service user as an individual, respecting their values, dignity, beliefs, preferences and needs according to the principles of good practice.

Understanding other people and yourself

Many illnesses and conditions can affect the mood and behaviour of the people to whom you provide care, such as:

- Pain
- Frustration
- Medication
- Stress
- Loneliness
- Sadness or grief
- Depression
- Fear

You must always remember to be patient when you are responding to someone whose behaviour you might (in your usual daily life) find rude or upsetting. Always think how you would like to be treated if you were unwell, upset or angry.

Talking and listening

Communication is fundamental to all our lives, enabling us to express what we want and fulfill our need to interact with other people.

Good communication is at the heart of good care. By talking with and listening to service users you will understand more about them as individuals – including their personalities, their backgrounds and the things they like and dislike, as well as their support needs. In turn, this will help you to provide care in a way that is acceptable to the service user.

Think about how you communicate and how this might affect the way you work with service users. Do you talk quickly or slowly? Do you look directly at people when you speak to them? What does your body language say? How do you check whether a service user understands you? Do you give people a chance to reply? You might need to change some of your own behaviours to make sure people can understand you or to ensure that they feel they are being listened to.

- Communicate with service users at their pace and in a style that suits them. A person's personality, background or culture may be a factor in the way you communicate with them.

- Depending on the service user's needs, you may need to learn new ways of communicating, such as using electronic or mechanical communication aids.

- If you work with service users who have sensory impairment (problems with their vision, hearing etc), you may need to use different communication techniques. There is more information about this in *Chapter 8 – The human body and health*.

- Some people can find it particularly difficult to find the right words for things – for example those with dysphasia (see *Chapter 10 – Common conditions*) or dementia (see *Chapter 11 – Supporting people with dementia*). Allow people time to say what they want to say, and try to avoid finishing people's sentences for them, as this can lead to misunderstandings and can be very frustrating for the service user.

- Recognise the needs of service users who don't speak English as a first language.

Going into a person's home

- Before you visit a service user, make sure you know how you will get into their home – for example, whether there is a door entry system, whether the service user is able to come to the door or whether you need a code for a key safe.

- When you meet someone for the first time, find out how they would like to be addressed. Be respectful and friendly and first greet the service user as Mr …, Mrs … or Ms … These titles should be used until you are given permission to call them by another name.

- Every time you arrive, make sure the service user knows you are there, who you are and what you will be doing while you are there. This is particularly important if they have problems with their sight or hearing, if they have memory problems, or if you let yourself into the house without the service user coming to the door. This is also important, as a service user may have a number of different people calling in during the day.

- Your agency or employer will give you an ID card. Always take it with you and be prepared to show it if someone asks.

- Saying "goodbye" is as important as saying "hello". Make sure the service user knows when you are leaving.

- If you can't get into the person's home for some reason, report this to your supervisor straight away and take instructions about what to do next. It is absolutely vital that you do not just leave because the person does not answer.

- Your employer will have a written policy, which you should have read and understood before you work on your own.

Time-sheets and electronic monitoring systems

As a careworker you will probably have to work a rota when visiting service users, and keep a record of the time you arrive and leave their homes. Some organisations use a time-sheet, and others use an electronic monitoring system. In the latter case careworkers keep the office informed of their movements by using a mobile phone or smart device, or by calling a Freephone number from the service user's phone when they arrive and leave.

Enabling service users to make choices

In your role, you will meet many different service users who have different needs and preferences. It is important that everyone working in social care puts the person and their preference at the centre of the care they provide. This is known as personalisation and means that services should be tailored to the needs and preferences of individuals. Throughout this book we return to this theme and the importance of providing care in a way that suits the individual service user.

When you are working with a service user, beware of the temptation to 'take over' and make decisions on their behalf. You will find different ways to understand your service users' preferences, such as:

- "Tell me what you'd like me to do today."

- "Would you like me to ...?"

- "I think I'll ... Is that alright?"

- "It looks to me as though ... needs doing. What do you think?"

- "I can see ... Can you? I think it would be a good idea to ..., don't you?"

- "Is there anything that you've noticed that needs doing?"

- "Today is Monday. What is today's programme?"

- "Do you think you'd like it if I ...?"

- "There's ... in the kitchen. Is that what you would like to eat?"

Care plans and record keeping

All of your service users will have a care plan, usually kept at their home. The care plan describes the type of care they need and should also describe how they would like to receive it. The care plan will also describe what the service user wants to achieve, with your assistance, and the outcomes that are important to them. The outcomes will be personal, may change over time and could be about achieving something new or maintaining a current skill or ability.

The care plan will also contain relevant information about risk assessment and how to avoid hazards while you work. It's important that you're familiar with the care plan so you can provide care in the way the service user prefers.

The care plan will usually have a daily log attached. This is an important record and communication tool for you and your organisation, as well as the service user and their family. It is essential that you read the previous entry in the log so you are fully up-to-date with anything that needs to be done by you or communicated back to your manager. You also need to make an accurate record of your visit so that the next careworker or family member can see what happened. An accurate record can help your organisation observe changing needs and requirements of the service user to ensure they continue to get the best possible service.

Confidentiality and security

You are likely to find out a lot about the service users you visit regularly, including information about their health, their private lives and their finances. In order to maintain service users' privacy, you must not share any information about them except where it is necessary for your work.

Part of your job will involve keeping records about your visits to service users. How and where these records are kept will depend on your agency's policies and the requirements set out by regulatory bodies.

These records are confidential. In order to maintain service users' privacy, the information they contain should only be shared according to your agency's guidelines. Service users have the right to see their own records if they wish. Again, your agency will have a policy about this.

As you go about your work, take care to protect service users' privacy and make sure that information about them remains confidential.

- You may meet a service user's friends or neighbours during your visit, or when you are on your way in or out of the service user's home. Make sure you never gossip about the service user or share any private information about them.

- If you use social media such as Facebook or Twitter, make sure you don't mention anything about your work that could compromise the confidentiality of your service users.

- Your employer will have a policy on mobile phone use that will ban personal use of a mobile phone while providing care to a service user. Careworkers will also need to take care not to store personal information about service users on their own mobile phone. Where information is stored on a mobile phone provided for work purposes, it should be kept locked to prevent others from accessing the information stored on it.

- You may want to make notes about a service user as part of your coursework for a vocational qualification. If so, use a code (such as service user A, service user B etc) rather than using real names. Your course assessor will be able to give you more information about this.

- Never leave keys or confidential records in a car, or anywhere where they might be seen by someone else or stolen. If anything is stolen or lost, report it to your supervisor immediately.

- Follow your agency's procedures for entering service users' homes and take extreme care that service users' privacy and security are not put at risk.

Smoking in the home

You must not smoke in a service user's home. However, you may have to go into homes where a service user, or someone else who lives in the home, is a smoker. Your employer has a duty to protect you from the health risks associated with breathing in other people's smoke. See *Chapter 5 – Health and safety at work* for more information.

Complaints and feedback

Service users and their family members or representatives have a right to make a complaint or comment about the service they receive, and to have these recorded or investigated where appropriate. To resolve complaints in a fair and open way, your employer will have procedures to follow. UKHCA also has a complaints procedure. Complaints can be referred to UKHCA under certain circumstances, if they cannot be resolved directly by the agency concerned.

Your agency may give you a copy of its complaints procedure. If a service user wants to use it, encourage and help them to follow the process.

Your employer is also likely to have a way of gathering the views of service users on a regular basis through surveys and reviews, for example. Service users may also make comments about the service to you and you should ensure that you pass these on to your agency.

Service users' families

Many of the service users you work with will live with one or more family members. A family member may provide the majority of the person's care. You may also be employed to enable the family carer to go out or have a break. This is known as "respite care".

It is important to build a good relationship with service users' families. Family members can help you in your work by providing information about the service user's background, their preferences and any recent changes in their health or wellbeing. They can also give you ideas about the best way to support the service user. This can be particularly useful if the service user finds it difficult to communicate because of an illness or disability.

Sometimes you won't be able to carry out a care task in the way the family carer prefers, because you are bound by rules and regulations that don't apply to the family carer. The family carer may find this frustrating so it is important to explain why you can't do things their way. Be courteous and sympathetic to their concerns.

It is important to recognise the positive contribution that family carers can make to your work, particularly where the service user is not able to express themselves. However, you also need to remember that you are there to provide care and support to the service user and their needs and preferences are most important. If there seems to be a conflict between the family carer and the service user, you may have a role in encouraging the family carer to support the person to do as much as they can for themselves and to make their own choices. See *Chapter 9 – Mental health*, for more information about mental capacity and helping service users to make choices.

Always talk to your supervisor if:

- Members of the family are concerned or unhappy about what you can or can't do.

- The actions or behaviour of a family member prevent you from carrying out your role properly.

- A family carer does anything that makes you concerned about the service user's welfare.

Maintaining appropriate relationships

Forming positive relationships with service users and their families is an important part of your job. However, your relationships with them should always be professional rather than personal. For example, you might tell a friend about your own personal problems, but it would not be appropriate to discuss them with a service user. Be aware of professional boundaries and avoid blurring them – for example, you should not visit service users at times other than when your employer has asked you to, even if you begin to feel that the service user or their family are becoming your friends.

Maintaining clear professional boundaries is an essential element of safeguarding service users from potential abuse. Following your employer's guidance on professional boundaries will also ensure you don't behave in ways that might be misinterpreted by other people.

See also *Chapter 19 – Self-expression and sexuality*, and *Chapter 22 – Household tasks and money management*.

Gifts from service users or their families

Sometimes a service user may want to give you a gift. In this situation, make sure you follow your agency's policy. You may be required to tactfully refuse all gifts, or there may be situations in which it is appropriate to accept a gift if it is of low monetary value. You may be required to report any gifts you accept. These guidelines are in place to safeguard service users by helping to prevent a careworker from being able to gain inappropriately from them. By following the guidelines you are also protecting yourself from potential claims that you are taking advantage of a service user. Also see *Chapter 22 – Household tasks and money management*.

Recognising abuse and neglect

As a careworker, your role is to look after the best interests of service users. To do this, you need to know about the possible signs of abuse and what you should do if you think a service user is being abused, neglected or mistreated.

The secretive nature of abuse and the shame that victims sometimes feel, can mean that abusive situations can continue over long periods of time. It is important that those caring for vulnerable adults are aware of, and are vigilant to, what may be signs of abuse. These can include:

• Frequent or unexplained injuries

• Untreated injuries and medical problems

• Being emotionally upset and agitated

• Inconsistency or difficulty in accounting for the cause of injuries

• The service user not being allowed to speak for themselves

• Poor personal hygiene, unchanged bedding and/or unsuitable clothing for the conditions or the environment

• Untreated or long-standing pressure sores that do not heal

• Unexplained weight loss or gain, or evidence of dehydration such as poor skin condition and/or frequent urinary infections

- The service user appearing withdrawn, depressed, having irregular sleep patterns, low self-esteem, fearfulness, agitation, or loss of appetite

- Abrupt or unexplainable changes to bank accounts or wills.

If you become concerned that one of your service users is being abused, you need to raise these concerns with your supervisor as soon as possible. You will need to follow your company policy on reporting abuse and your supervisor will be able to help you through that.

If for any reason you're unable to report the issue to your own organisation you can contact the relevant care regulator (See *Chapter 2 – Standards and regulations in the homecare sector*, for details).

Surveillance by webcam or CCTV

Service users and their families are increasingly using webcams or CCTV for surveillance purposes in the home. This is a useful tool if a service user is alone for long periods, or has a tendency to fall or wander. Careworkers should expect to encounter surveillance equipment in the course of their work, and may indeed be videoed while they are working. If you are uncomfortable with this, you should discuss this with your manager. It is legal for service users and their families to use such equipment *without* informing the homecare organisation. However, whether you are being recorded or not, you should work at all times as though your actions could be seen by somebody else.

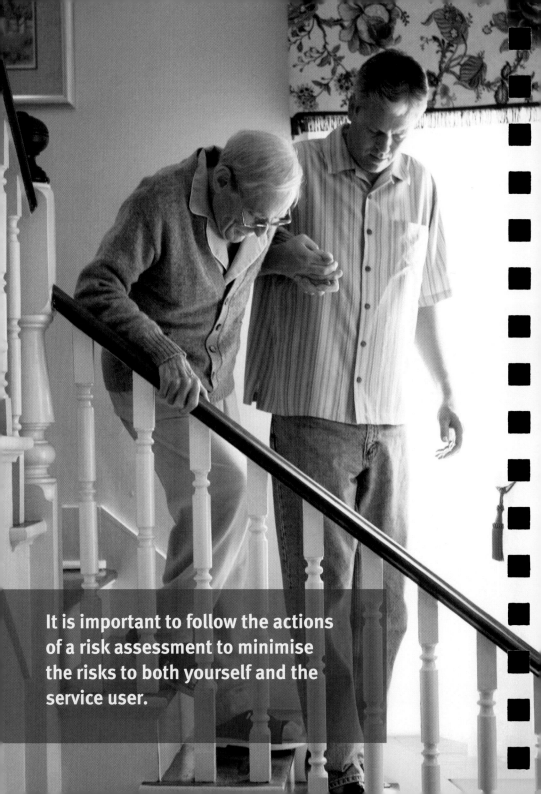

It is important to follow the actions of a risk assessment to minimise the risks to both yourself and the service user.

5   Health and safety at work

Both you and your employer have a legal responsibility to look after your health, safety and welfare while you are at work. As an employee, you also have responsibilities for your own safety and for the welfare of service users.

The rules about health and safety are outlined in the Health and Safety at Work Act 1974, and in detailed regulations such as the Management of Health and Safety at Work Regulations 1999.

Your employer's responsibilities

Your employer should have health and safety policies and procedures in place, which set out the things they will do to avoid risks to your health and safety, and that of others, while you are at work.

Policies and procedures should be available for all aspects of your work, including:

* Reporting accidents and injuries
* Moving and handling
* Infection control
* Using hazardous substances
* Working on your own – 'lone working'.

Your employer should provide you with, or give you access to, the organisation's health and safety policies and procedures. Make sure you read them and understand what they mean for you. Your employer should provide relevant training and guidance to help you to follow the policies and procedures that apply to your work.

All employers are required by law to assess the risks that their employees face in the workplace. In the case of homecare, the workplace usually means service users' homes. An assessment should identify significant risks and what needs to be done to reduce the risks. It is important to follow the actions identified in a risk assessment to minimise the risks to both yourself and the service user. You must also inform your supervisor whenever you think there is a new risk or a change to an existing risk.

Sometimes the agency may be asked to provide a service urgently, and there may not be enough time to carry out a risk assessment before you visit a person's home. In these situations, your employer should let you know that no assessment has yet been carried out. You should take special care and inform your supervisor immediately if you think there is any risk to you or to the service user.

Your responsibilities

As a careworker, you must take responsibility for your health and safety in the workplace, and the wellbeing of those around you.

- Always follow your agency's health and safety policies and procedures. Work in accordance with the instructions and training you have received on health and safety.

- Use equipment or protective clothing provided by your employer.

- Look out for potential risks or hazards and report them to your supervisor.

- If you think that your working conditions have changed in a way that increases the risk to your health and safety or that of the service user, inform your supervisor so that the situation can be reassessed.

Employed or self-employed careworkers

Careworkers are usually:

- employed by a homecare provider
- employed by a service user or
- self-employed.

This handbook assumes that the careworker is employed by the homecare provider. Much of the information it contains is relevant to all types of careworker, but the balance of responsibilities will vary. For example, where a service user employs a careworker they assume the responsibilities of an employer, including for health and safety. The precise differences between the types of arrangement are beyond the scope of this handbook.

Lone working

Most careworkers work on their own, which can make them more vulnerable to some types of health and safety risk. For example, you might have to travel in isolated or unlit areas, or deal with a service user or relative who is behaving aggressively. Employers should take lone working into account when carrying out risk assessments, and should make sure that you have regular supervision and training. Your employer or agency will have systems in place to minimise the risks of lone working. These might include:

- An on-call system so that careworkers can make contact with someone outside of normal working hours if necessary.

- A system where careworkers phone in to the office at set times or at the end of their shift.

- A 'buddy' system whereby two lone careworkers meet up together at certain times of day.

- Lone worker safety equipment, for example, a personal safety alarm or first aid box if you are working in remote areas.

It is important to follow the procedures that your agency or employer has put in place to protect your health and safety.

If you feel uncomfortable, threatened or unsafe in someone's home, leave as soon as you can and contact your agency for advice or help.

Chemicals and dangerous substances

Most of the household products that you use in a service user's home will not pose a significant risk to you or the service user, as long as the products are used and stored in line with manufacturers' instructions.

If you need to use a substance that is not a normal household product, consult your employer. They should make sure you have the information you need about how to use it and any precautions you should take, such as wearing gloves.

Never mix products together, even if you think that they are similar and they perform similar functions – for example bleach and some toilet cleaners. Mixing products together can produce dangerous fumes.

Make sure all products are kept in their original containers. If you are not sure what is in a container or if you can't read the instructions, do not use it. Take special care when storing substances in the home of a service user who is blind or partially sighted. Also, remember that someone who has lost their sense of smell may find it more difficult to identify substances.

Electricity

There are three main hazards associated with electricity.

1. Contact with live parts can cause shock and burns (normal mains voltage can kill).

2. Electrical faults can cause fires.

3. Electricity could be the source of ignition in an explosive atmosphere, for example, if there is a gas leak or there is medical oxygen present.

If you see that an electrical appliance in a service user's home is damaged or in a poor state of repair, do not use it and tell the service user and your employer about it.

In an emergency you may need to know where to find the main electricity switch in your service users' homes. If electrical equipment gives off an unusual smell, appears to be overheating or is sparking, turn the electricity off at the main switch first, and then unplug the appliance.

If you are in any doubt about the safety of any electrical item, do not use it until it has been checked by someone who is qualified to do so.

Remember:

- To turn off fully any electrical appliances that don't need to be switched on all the time, with the service user's agreement.

- Not to use any electrical appliances in the bathroom, apart from those that are specially wired in.

- To use a residual current device (RCD) (also known as a circuit breaker) in service users' homes if your agency has provided you with one. RCDs are safety devices that switch off electricity automatically if there is a fault. It is used like an adapter – the RCD plugs into a normal socket, and then the appliance is plugged into the RCD.

Fire

Heat, fuel (anything that burns) and oxygen are needed to start a fire – and these are all common in the average home. It is important to keep sources of heat and fuel apart. Sources of heat include radiators, electrical appliances, chemical reactions (when two substances mix together, intentionally or unintentionally), sunlight (especially when focused through glass) and friction (created when two materials or objects rub against each other). Paper, fabrics, furniture, cushions or bedclothes can all become fuel, and oxygen is in the surrounding air.

It is therefore important to prevent any chance of a fire and to ensure that fire prevention equipment is working, particularly as your service users may have difficulty noticing a fire, or leaving their home if a fire starts.

- Make sure clothes are not left to dry on fire guards or on electric heaters, and that tea towels are not hung to dry on the cooker.

- Clothes should not be hung where they trail over radiators.

- Smoke alarms should be tested regularly and the batteries replaced when necessary.

- Domestic fire extinguishers should be serviced once a year by a qualified engineer. (Fire blankets do not need servicing.)

Gas

Where a service user has a gas supply in their home, check that the gas fires, cookers and ovens are off when they are not in use, especially if the service user is not very mobile or has memory problems. In an emergency you may need to know where the main gas valve is in order to turn it off.

Find out the position of any alarms, such as carbon monoxide detectors or smoke alarms, and notify your organisation if you suspect they are not working.

If you arrive at someone's home and find that a gas burner is on but unlit, turn off the burner and open the windows immediately to allow the gas to escape. If there is a strong smell of gas, evacuate with the service user if possible and notify your supervisor immediately, who will then contact the emergency gas number to report it.

Report events such as unlit gas burners to your supervisor. This will enable the agency to take the necessary steps to ensure the health and safety of the service user and others.

If a service user lives in a rented home (either council or private), their landlord is responsible for carrying out regular gas safety checks.

Water

Water can be a hazard because it can make floors and surfaces slippery and can be difficult to see. It can also cause damage to other things in the home.

- Always mop up any water that has been spilled on bathroom, lavatory or kitchen floors.

- If you notice a leaking appliance or device you should notify your organisation. Turn off the water supply if you know how to do this.

- In an emergency you may need to know where the stopcock or mains tap is in the houses you visit, so that you can turn off the main water supply if there is a leak or flood. Stopcocks are often, but not always, located under the kitchen sink.

In case of emergency

IF YOU NEED THE POLICE, AN AMBULANCE, THE FIRE BRIGADE OR THE COASTGUARD, CALL 999

Household hazards

Be on the lookout for potential hazards as you go about your work so that problems can be fixed before they cause any harm. If you think something presents a health and safety risk, report it to your supervisor.

Hazards around the home might include:

- Wrinkled carpets or rugs, or stair carpets that are not firmly fixed.

- Slippery floors.

- Uneven or damaged steps or stairs.

- Poor lighting.

- Walking sticks and zimmer frames without ferrules (non-slip tips), which may become unsteady.

- Steam from pans or kettles, or unsteady saucepans.

- Sharp or rough objects.

- Chipped or cracked glass or crockery.

- Products that do not have a label, or are wrongly labelled.

- Products that are stored in unsuitable containers.

Infection control

It is essential to protect yourself and service users against infections (also see *Chapter 10 – Common health conditions*). This means following some simple rules.

- Follow your agency's policy and guidance on infection control.

- Wash your hands well with soap and warm water, and dry them thoroughly, using disposable paper towels or a clean hand towel. Wash your hands:

  - Before and after each of your visits to service users.
  - After contact with bodily fluids or secretions.
  - After handling soiled or contaminated equipment, clothes or bedding.
  - Before eating, drinking or handling food.
  - After using the toilet.
  - After touching animals, or animal foods.

- If soap, water or towels are not available, your employer may provide you with a liquid hand wash or gel.

- If you have cuts or grazes on your hands, cover them with a waterproof dressing.

- Use disposable waterproof gloves and aprons when dealing with spillages of bodily fluids or carrying out any procedures that involve contact with open wounds or broken skin. Used gloves and aprons should be taken off correctly and should be disposed of with the usual household waste.

- Clean supplies or equipment thoroughly if taking them from one person's home into another's.

- Clean equipment such as commodes thoroughly with detergent and hot water after use.

- If changing a service user's bedding, try to avoid creating dust. Don't shake out sheets and bedding and don't hug it to you when taking it to the washing machine.

- Clothes and bedding should be machine washed. It is fine to use a normal household washing machine on the hot wash setting.

- If clothes or bed-linen are soiled with faeces, use disposable gloves and paper towels to remove as much as possible before putting them in the washing machine.

- Keep your fingernails short and clean and free from nail varnish and false nails.

- Tie your hair back when cooking and working closely with service users.

- Cough or sneeze into a tissue or handkerchief and wash your hands straight afterwards.

If a service user or colleague has an infectious disease that could put you at risk, discuss this with your supervisor. For example, shingles and chicken pox are caused by the same virus, so if a service user or colleague has shingles and you have never had chicken pox, there is a possibility you could contract chicken pox from contact with that person.

If a careworker has a bout of diarrhoea and/or vomiting they should not prepare food for at least 48 hours after the sickness has stopped.

Food Hygiene

Good hygiene practices in relation to storing and preparing food will reduce the risk of infections caused by food.

- Wash fresh fruit or vegetables thoroughly, even organic produce.

- Keep raw and cooked food separate and don't use the same utensils and equipment for both without thoroughly washing these in between.

- Store food correctly.

- Cook food at the correct temperature, for the correct length of time particularly if reheating food; food cooked at the wrong temperature could encourage bacteria to grow.

- Clear up any spillages straight away.

See *Chapter 17 – Food and nutrition*, for more information.

Medicines

Your work may involve the supervision of service users when they need to take medicines or apply creams or lotions. If so, it is essential to understand and follow your agency's policies and procedures on this. See *Chapter 16 – Helping service users with medication*, for more detailed information.

Moving and handling

It is important for your own health and safety to follow the guidance on moving and handling. See *Chapter 6 – Helping service users to move*, for more detailed information.

Smoking – in service users' homes

Smoking is banned in almost all workplaces. However the smoking ban does not apply to service users' own homes. If a service user or someone who lives with them is a smoker, there is a risk that you may be exposed to passive smoking (breathing in someone else's smoke) while you are at work.

Your employer has a responsibility to ensure that you are adequately protected from the risk of passive smoking. They must balance this with the right of the service user to smoke in their own home if they wish.

Your employer should have a policy in place to minimise the risk to staff. This may include measures such as:

- Asking service users who smoke to agree not to smoke shortly before the careworker arrives and when they are present.

- Making sure a careworker doesn't have to visit two or more houses in succession where there is likely to be smoke.

- Identifying staff who have conditions that may be worsened by exposure to smoke, such as asthma or chronic bronchitis, and those who may be at higher risk of harm, such as pregnant women.

If you are concerned about the risk of passive smoking in a particular service user's home, discuss the situation with your supervisor. Careworkers should never smoke in any service user's home, even if the service user or their family say it is alright to do so.

Smoking – in cars used for work

The law requires that pool cars or company cars that are used by more than one person must be smoke-free. This does not apply to workers who use a car that is 'primarily for the private purposes of the person who owns it'. However if you use your own car for work, your employer or agency may have a policy that requires you to keep it smoke-free, particularly if you use it to transport other staff or service users. Check your employer's policy to find out how it affects you.

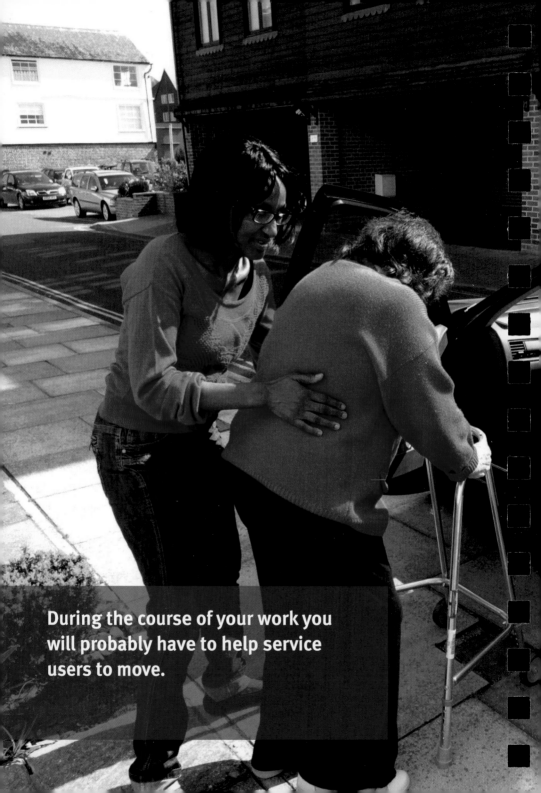

During the course of your work you will probably have to help service users to move.

6   Helping service users to move

During the course of your work you will probably have to help service users to move – for example, to help them get out of bed and into a chair, or to use the bathroom. Your employer has a responsibility to make sure that you have the training, help, equipment and space to do this in a way that reduces the risk of injury to the service user, yourself or others.

As a careworker you also have a responsibility for your own health and safety and that of others, so it is vital to follow safe systems of working and inform your supervisor if there are any changes that affect your ability to move a service user.

Managing risk – employers' and careworkers' responsibilities

Where it is necessary to help a service user to move, your employer is responsible for carrying out a risk assessment. The risk assessment must be recorded as part of the service user's care plan. It should offer clear instructions on how the service user can be safely moved, taking into account the following points:

- The task to be carried out
- Information about the service user
- The environment (the working area)
- The careworker's ability to carry out the task

All risk assessments must be regularly reviewed. A review should also take place if the handling situation changes, reports show the situation is proving difficult, or if there is an accident.

It is your responsibility to:

- Follow safe ways of working as identified in training or by your supervisor.

- Make proper use of the equipment provided and tell your supervisor if it is broken or unsafe to use, or if you do not know how to use it.

- Let your supervisor know if there is a change in the service user's condition that could affect their safety or the safety of careworkers.

- Tell your supervisor if there is a change in your own health that affects your ability to move service users.

Your agency will have policies and procedures covering these requirements and should provide you with proper training in handling and moving service users during your induction. This chapter is intended to offer a helpful reminder.

Looking after your back

Think about ways of carrying out tasks that avoid bending your back, twisting or maintaining a static stooped position for any length of time.

Things to take into account before moving someone

Every service user's situation is different, and may vary from day to day, or even hour to hour. The service user handling assessment will have taken various factors into account to identify the tasks required and whether there are any additional needs, such as a hoist or another careworker. You must also take into account the following points:

For the service user

- Particular problems or conditions the service user may have, such as arthritis or multiple sclerosis.

- Their size or shape – are they particularly tall, large or heavy? People who are overweight may sit or move in a different way to those of average weight, which could make a difference to the way you approach moving tasks.

- Their mental state – do they become confused or distressed easily?

- Can the service user help you to move them or follow prompts and instructions you give them?

- Posture – can the service user hold themselves upright?

- Sensory difficulties – can the person see or hear?

- Pressure areas – so that you can avoid friction or damage.

- Can the service user be moved without causing them pain?

For the working area

- Is there enough space to carry out the task safely?

- Are there obstacles in your way, especially things left on the floor?

- Furniture – is it large, heavy or awkward? Is it easy to move?

- Positioning – can you get behind the service user if you need to? How will you position the service user?

- Is there enough light?

- Are there different floor levels and surfaces to take into account?

For yourself

Finally, are you able to carry out the task? You can't learn to move and handle service users just by reading a book – your employer will provide training. You may also be able to take advantage of other courses that are available. This chapter should support and remind you as you go about your work.

Principles of safe moving and handling

There is always an element of risk when moving a service user, but by following the guidelines you can help to keep yourself and the service user safe.

- Before you begin, think about the whole process and work out what you need to do from start to finish.

- Encourage the service user to be as independent as possible.

- Always bend at the knee, not the waist. This allows your thigh and buttock muscles to do the work rather than putting all the pressure on your back.

- Make a stable base with your feet – ideally a medium stride apart, no wider than your shoulders.

- If working on a bed, stand with one knee on the bed to create a stable base.

- Keep as close as possible to the service user.

- Avoid twisting or jerking movements.

- Avoid twisting and bending at the same time.

- Always have your lead foot facing in the direction you are moving in to avoid twisting your back.

- Avoid stooping for long periods.

- Take your time and coordinate all movements and make sure everyone knows what to do and when to do it. Use clear, precise instructions, for example, "ready, steady" and then the action required such as "stand" or "slide".

- Take extra care when helping a service user with stairs. Giving physical support to someone going up or down stairs could pose a risk to yourself or the service user. If the service user needs physical support to manage stairs, talk to your supervisor about how best their needs can be met.

- Always wear flat shoes and clothes that let you move freely. Remove sharp objects such as jewellery.

- Do not try to move anyone who is pulling back or resisting the move.

- Never allow the service user to put their arms around your neck.

- All moves that include holding a service user's armpits are no longer considered safe.

- If you are in any doubt about your ability to move someone safely, do not try it. If you have any problems carrying out moves, talk to your supervisor about them.

And remember the golden rule: you should never lift most, or all, of a service user's weight.

Aids and adaptations

You may be required to use aids in the moving and handling of your service users. Where this is the case your employer will have given you training on how they should be used based on the manufacturer's instructions. These will also indicate how often they should be maintained and your organisation will ensure that this takes place. If you notice any problems or defects with equipment that you are required to use you should report them to your supervisor immediately.

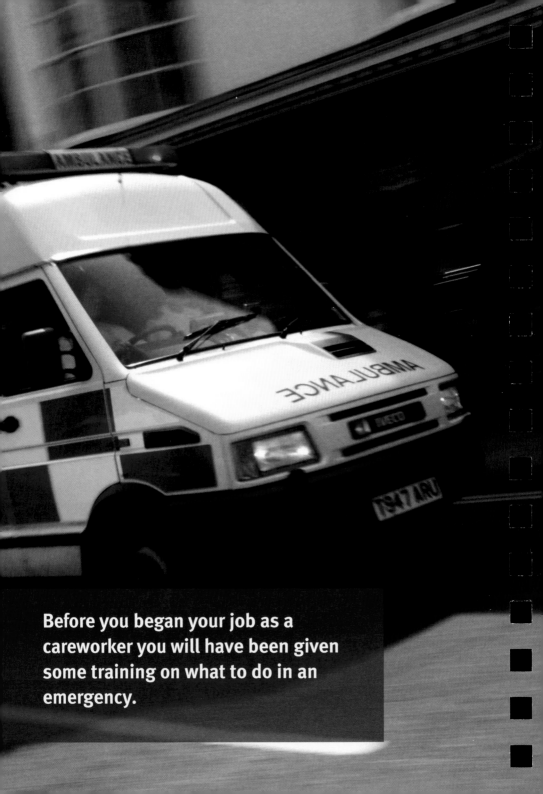

Before you began your job as a careworker you will have been given some training on what to do in an emergency.

7   What to do in an emergency

Before you began your job as a careworker you will have been given some training on what to do in an emergency. You should also have been made aware of your employer's policies and procedures relating to emergency situations. You should look at these again from time to time to refresh your memory.

The following instructions are set out as briefly as possible in case you need to refer to them in an emergency.

Fire

• In the event of a fire, raise the alarm.

• Dial 999 and ask for the fire brigade, giving clear instructions about the location of the fire.

• If appropriate, help the service user to leave the premises if it is safe to do so.

• If safe to do so, close windows and doors to prevent fire and smoke spreading.

• It is usually safer to leave a building than tackle a fire yourself.

• Do not re-enter a building to collect personal belongings.

• Do not return to the building until the fire brigade has confirmed it is safe to do so.

• Report the incident to your supervisor as soon as it is safe to do so.

• Keep calm and reassure the service user.

Water leak or flooding

- Put a bucket or bowl underneath the flow of water if possible.

- Turn off the stopcock (the tap that controls the mains water supply to the flat or house) to cut off the water supply.

- If water is coming from the main water tank in the house, leave the bath tap running. If the stopcock has been turned off, the water in the tank will run out, temporarily stopping the leak or flood.

- Telephone your office or the emergency number of the water company that supplies water in the service user's area, if you know it.

- Use towels or other absorbent materials to mop up water – it is best to use things made of natural fibres, as man-made fibres are not very absorbent.

- Keep calm and reassure the service user.

Gas or fumes

- Gas is explosive and harmful to breathe. If there is a strong smell of gas, you should evacuate the building and raise the alarm.

- If you are able, open windows to let gases or fumes escape.

- Turn off any fires or cookers and DO NOT LIGHT matches, candles, tapers, cigarette lighters or anything else which could cause the gas to ignite.

- Turn off the main gas supply where it enters the house or flat.

- Do not turn on/off any electrical switches or use your mobile phone on the premises.

- If there are any electrical security entry phones/locks, please open door manually.

- Telephone the gas emergency number 0800 111 999.

- Telephone your office as soon as it is safe to do so.

- Try to identify the source of any fumes that are not related to the gas supply, if it is safe to do so.

- If the service user is having difficulty breathing, or is coughing, hold a damp cloth across their nose and mouth – do the same for yourself if needed.

- If the fumes continue to be a problem, consider going outside.

- Inform your supervisor as soon as it is safe to do so.

Electric shock

- DO NOT TOUCH a person if they are in contact with the electrical supply.

- Turn off the electricity supply at the mains.

- If you can't turn off the electricity, stand on a dry rubber mat, dry wooden block or book (such as a telephone directory) and use a wooden broom handle or something similar to push the person's limbs away from the electrical supply. NEVER USE ANYTHING METAL.

- Dial 999 for an ambulance.

- Treat the person for shock (see page 61).

- Inform your supervisor as soon as it is safe to do so.

Health-related emergencies

Is the person having a heart attack?

Does the service user have:

- severe chest pains?
- breathlessness?
- sudden faintness or giddiness?
- very pale or grey skin?
- blue lips?
- rapid pulse?

If so:

- dial 999 for an ambulance immediately

- sit the person up, if possible, with their knees bent (the 'W' position)

- give the person a 300mg aspirin tablet to chew slowly (unless there is a reason not to, for example, they are allergic to it). This will be recorded in the service user's care plan.

- keep the service user warm

- give plenty of reassurance.

Has the person collapsed, are they unconscious?

Tilt the head back, lift and hold the chin to keep their airway open.

Check if the person is breathing –

- Is their chest moving?
- Can you hear them breathing?
- Can you feel their breath?

If the person is breathing:

- Place the person on their side in the recovery position if this can be done safely.

- Dial 999 for an ambulance.

- Keep the person warm.

- Regularly check that they are still breathing.

- Administer first aid if you have been trained and in line with your organisation's policies.

If the person is not breathing:

- Dial 999 for an ambulance.

- Begin chest compressions.

- Using the heel of your hand only push down hard and fast in the middle of the chest at a rate of 100-120 per minute.

- Keep pushing and releasing at a regular rate until the ambulance arrives.

NOTE: Only administer CPR if you have previously received appropriate training.

Has the person had a stroke?

Remember the FAST guide:

- **F**ace – Has their face fallen on one side? Can they smile?
- **A**rms – Can they raise both arms and keep them there?
- **S**peech – Is their speech slurred?
- **T**ime – Time to call 999 for emergency help if you see any single one of these signs.

Is the person bleeding from a wound?

- Dial 999 for an ambulance if the wound is serious.

- If the wound is on an arm or leg, apply pressure by placing a clean, dry pad over the wound.

- If there is glass or another foreign body sticking out of the wound, put a pad round the wound.

- Raise the limb so that it is higher than the rest of the body, if this will not cause further harm.

- If the bleeding is very heavy, apply pressure to the limb between the wound and the heart.

Is the person choking – is their airway blocked?

Encourage the person to cough, to try and remove the obstruction. If this fails follow the instructions below:

Back blows

- Bend the person forward.

- Use the heel of your hand to give up to five sharp blows between the person's shoulder blades in an upward direction.

- Check between blows to see if the blockage has cleared.

If this does not remove the obstruction:

Abdominal thrusts

- Stand behind the person.

- Put your arms around their waist.

- Make a fist with one hand and place it between the navel and the bottom of the rib cage.

- Grasp your fist with your other hand and pull sharply inwards and upwards.

- Repeat this up to five times rechecking the mouth to see if the blockage has cleared.

If the person's airway is still blocked

- Repeat the cycle of 5 back blows and 5 abdominal thrusts twice and if still not clear:

- Dial 999 for an ambulance.

- Continue the sequence until the ambulance arrives, the obstruction is cleared or the person loses consciousness.

NOTE: This technique should not be used on anyone who is under one year old, pregnant or obese.

Abdominal thrusts can cause injury, you must make sure the person is checked by a medical professional afterwards, to make sure they have not been injured and that the obstruction has completely cleared.

Has the person been burned or scalded?

- Depending on which part of the person's body is burned, run cool water over the burn for at least 10 minutes.

- While cooling the burn, carefully remove any clothing or jewellery, unless it is attached to the skin.

- Seek medical advice urgently, including calling 999 for serious burns or scalds.

- Keep the person warm, using blankets or layers of clothing on parts of the body that are not injured, to prevent the person becoming dangerously cold.

- Cover the burn lengthways with strips of cling film, or if the burn is on a hand or foot, a clean plastic bag. If no plastic film is available, use a sterile dressing. Don't use anything fluffy.

- DO NOT apply ice, creams, ointments or fats (such as butter) to the burn or surrounding area.

- DO NOT burst blisters.

Is the person in shock?

Does the service user have, or are they developing some or all of the following signs:

- a rapid pulse?

- pale, grey skin? (When pressed, does an earlobe or fingernail not regain its colour straight away?)

- cold, clammy skin?

- weakness, dizziness or nausea (feeling sick)?

- rapid, shallow breathing?

If so:

- dial 999 for an ambulance

- help the person to lie down

- raise and support their legs

- loosen any tight clothing they may be wearing

- keep the person warm but do not apply direct heat, such as a hot water bottle

- reassure the person and let them know that help is on its way

- be prepared to resuscitate them if their condition gets worse and if you are trained to do so

- DO NOT let the person move unnecessarily

- DO NOT give them any food or drink

Does the person have a broken bone?

- Is the person in extreme pain?

- Has part of their body swelled up?

- Is there bone sticking out from a wound?

- Is the person unable to move the affected area?

If so:

- dial 999 for an ambulance.

- do not move the person – or if they are conscious, encourage them to keep still.

- keep the person warm.

- support the injured limb until help arrives.

- look out for signs of shock (see previous page).

- DO NOT give the person anything to eat or drink.

Has the person swallowed something poisonous?

- Dial 999 for an ambulance and, if you can, tell the ambulance service what type of substance the person has swallowed.

- Keep packaging or bottles and show them to the emergency services when they arrive.

- Check the person's breathing.

- Check their pulse.

- Keep the person warm and still.

- DO NOT give them anything to eat or drink, and DO NOT try to make them sick.

Is the person unconscious?

- Check the person's mouth for vomit or any other possible blockage.

- Check for any false teeth and whether or not they are in position. If not, remove them.

- Put the person into the recovery position.

Does the person have asthma?

Find out who to contact if the person has an asthma attack and what medication they can take to relieve an attack. You may be able to find this out from the person's GP or from their care plan.

As a general rule, if a person has an asthma attack, encourage them to:

- take one or two puffs of reliever treatment (via an inhaler) immediately

- sit down or sit, well-supported in bed and take slow, steady breaths

If this does not help:

- the person should continue to use their inhaler, as described on the packaging

- if the attack continues, dial 999 for an ambulance

- DO NOT let the person lie down

After an emergency asthma attack, encourage the person to make an appointment with their GP or asthma nurse for a review.

Does the person have diabetes?

If the service user is showing some of the following symptoms they may be suffering from hypoglycaemia (a "hypo") caused by low blood sugar.

Is the service user:

- Sweating?
- Feeling tired, weak or fatigued?
- Feeling dizzy?
- Looking pale?
- Hungry?
- Showing a higher pulse rate than normal?
- Having palpitations (irregular heartbeat)?
- Reporting blurred vision or tingling lips?
- Unable to concentrate?
- Sleepy or slow to respond to conversation?
- Anxious, irritable or showing a mood change?
- Confused, or slow or slurred speech?
- Shaking?
- Losing consciousness?

If the service user is able to eat safely, IMMEDIATELY give them short-acting carbohydrates such as:

- a glass of fruit juice.
- a glass of glucose drink/drink containing sugar.
- three or more glucose tablets.
- five sweets, such as barley sugars.
- chocolate.

The exact amount will vary from person to person and will depend on the circumstances.

After giving the person short-acting carbohydrates, follow this with food containing longer-acting carbohydrates. This could be one of the following:

- a sandwich
- fruit
- biscuits and milk
- a bowl of cereal
- the next meal, if it is due

If the service user is UNCONSCIOUS:

- Put the person in the recovery position and call 999

Have you arrived and found that a service user has died?

- Dial 999 to call the emergency services.

- Ensure that the emergency services have any relevant information.

- Report the death to your agency.

- Do not touch or move the body unless instructed.

Dealing with abusive, violent or aggressive behaviour

- Keep calm.
- Don't argue.
- Keep your distance from the service user.
- Report the incident to your supervisor.

If a service user's behaviour is too aggressive for you to stay:

- Get between the person and the door.

- If they have taken hold of you, grab the person's thumbs to break their hold.

- Leave the room or the house if you are worried about your safety.

- Avoid using a personal alarm, which might shock the service user unless your safety is at risk.

- Report what has happened to your supervisor immediately.

- Call 999 if your safety is at immediate risk.

Implement any training you have been given on dealing with aggression and helping the service user become calm

What do to if a service user doesn't answer their door ('no reply' procedures)

- Your agency should have a policy and procedure for this situation, it is essential that you understand it and put it into practice.

- If a service user doesn't open their door, or does not appear to be at home when they are expected to be there, contact your agency immediately to find out if they have any information about where the person is. For example they may be in hospital or have gone to stay with a family member.

- If the agency does not have any information to suggest that the person is away, check his/her home if you can by looking through the windows and letterbox.

- If you can see that the person has collapsed or is in difficulties, dial 999 and ask for the police (to gain access to the house) and an ambulance. Let your agency know what has happened.

- If you can't see whether the person is in the house, check with neighbours, caretakers, wardens or anyone else who might know where the person is. If you find out that the person is safe, report this to your agency straight away.

- If, after carrying out the above checks, you are still not sure where the person is, or are concerned about their safety or wellbeing, contact your supervisor immediately so that your agency can take further action. You should not leave the home until you are certain where the service user is, or you are told to do so by your supervisor.

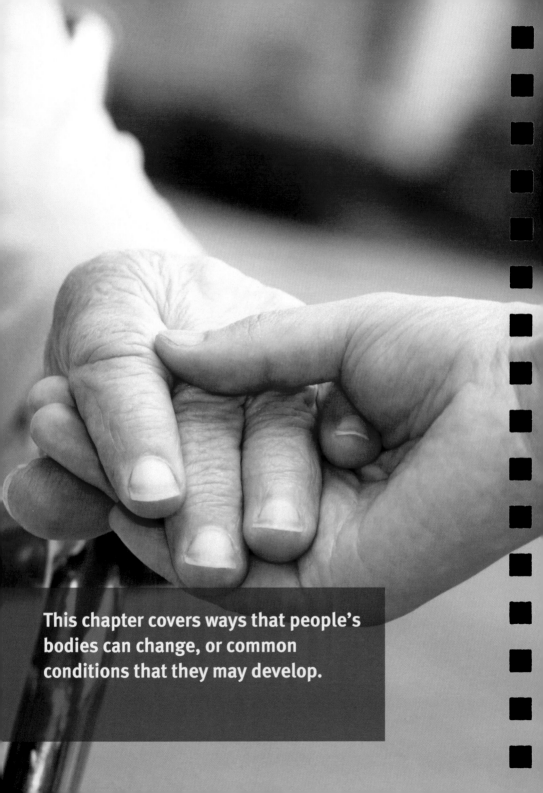

This chapter covers ways that people's bodies can change, or common conditions that they may develop.

8   The human body and health

This chapter describes the parts and systems of the human body. It describes how people's bodies can change, mainly as a result of getting older, but also because of general wear and tear, accidents, disease and the effects of disabilities, medical treatments and lifestyles.

Each section describes:

- What each part of the body does and sometimes, in simple terms, how it works.

- Ways that people's bodies can change, or common conditions that they may develop (mainly as a result of ageing).

- What this means for service users.

- What you should look out for and how you can help.

The skeleton, muscles and skin

The skeleton, along with the muscles and tendons that are attached to it, keep us upright and enable us to move. The skin provides a waterproof and infection-proof covering for the body.

What happens

- A person's bones may become brittle, which means they can break more easily. This condition, called osteoporosis, is more common in women than men.

- The discs between the bones of a person's spine may lose their water content or may become damaged. This can cause the spine to shrink or become curved and can cause pain and difficulty in moving.

- A person's joints can become misshapen because of diseases such as arthritis. This may mean the person cannot move their joints easily or quickly, and moving them becomes painful.

- A person's muscles may become less effective (or 'waste') because they don't use them very much or because they aren't getting enough nourishment in their diet. Some health conditions might mean that the person's muscles don't receive messages from the brain.

- As a person gets older, their skin is likely to become drier and thinner.

What this means for the service user

- Service users might become over-cautious because they are worried about breaking a bone. This can mean that they become less active.

- A lack of flexibility in the joints may mean that service users cannot move or bend easily. They might find it painful to move.

- It might be difficult or impossible for a service user to turn to look at someone.

- A service user's reactions might be delayed, or they may not be able to make the movements they want to make.

- The service user might find it difficult to hold or grip things. This means they could be more likely to drop things, or find it hard to do up buttons or hold a pen.

- A service user's skin could become cracked, sore or flaky.

- Even small cuts or grazes (particularly on a person's shin) can develop into ulcers.

- If a service user sits or lies in one position for a length of time, the pressure on one area of their body can lead to pressure sores.

What you can do

- Be firm but gentle when helping service users to move.

- Help to give the service user prescribed medication for pain relief if required to do so (see *Chapter 16 – Helping service users with medication*).

- Help the service user to sit or lie in a position that is comfortable and safe, using cushions, aids and other supports as necessary. If in doubt, you should talk to your supervisor about getting some advice from a physiotherapist.

- Look out for any changes in service users' skin, especially over bony parts of the body such as elbows, buttocks and heels. A change of colour or swelling could mean that a pressure sore is developing. If you spot these signs, talk to your supervisor straight away as the person may need immediate treatment.

- If a service user is not very mobile, encourage and help them to change position at least every two hours to avoid continuous pressure on the same parts of the body.

- Give service users extra time to do things like answer the door.

- Make sure service users can easily reach the things they need often, such as a walking stick, reading glasses or fluids.

- Talk to your supervisor if you think equipment or aids, such as a walking frame, would help a service user.

- Remember not to move furniture that has been put in special places, such as a kitchen stool that enables a service user to work at the sink or a chair that they use as a walking aid.

- Talk to your supervisor about contacting utility providers (ie the gas, water, electricity and telephone companies) for special aids such as Braille cooker controls, telephone stands and bells, if you think they would help a service user.

- Be patient if a service user's reactions and movements are slow.

- Be prepared for a service user's grip to be surprisingly strong – they may over-compensate because they are worried about losing hold.

- Make sure that a service user who is not able to move on their own is not sitting in a draught or too close to a fire.

- If a service user's clothes no longer fit because their body shape has changed, or if they find it difficult to get dressed or to do up fastenings, talk to your supervisor about getting their clothes altered or buying new clothes. (See *Chapter 20 – Washing and dressing*, for more guidance on helping people to get dressed.)

- Encourage service users to use hand or body lotion if they have dry skin. A community nurse may be able to recommend a lotion or cream that is particularly suited to older skin.

- If a service user has dry lips, suggest that they use a lip salve or cream.

- Encourage service users to have a balanced diet (but check in case they have been advised not to eat certain foods for medical reasons).

Hands and feet

Some of the information above applies to hands and feet, but there are some additional things you can do to help service users to maintain healthy hands and feet:

- Take special care to dry between a person's toes after washing their feet.

- Check the service user's toenails and look out for any uncomfortable hard skin. If their toenails or feet need attention, DO NOT TRY TO DO THIS YOURSELF – instead talk to your supervisor about contacting a chiropodist. Check the service user's fingernails and help them with cutting or filing their nails if necessary.

- Suggest removing (and replacing) any socks or stockings that are restricting a service user's blood flow.

- A service user who often has cold hands might benefit from wearing fingerless gloves, which provide warmth and still enable a person to hold and grip things.

- Make sure you don't tie a person's shoelaces too tight, as this could restrict the blood flow to their feet.

- Encourage service users to wiggle their toes and ankles to give them a little exercise and help their circulation. Encourage foot and hand exercises, such as gripping and releasing a tennis ball, which help people to keep their fingers supple and their muscles active.

- Make a note of any abrasions, such as grazes, blisters or burns, and report these to your supervisor.

The digestive system

The digestive system includes the mouth, the stomach and intestines and organs such as the liver and pancreas. Together these parts of the body break down the food we eat so that we can absorb the nutrients. They also take away the waste products. The digestive system processes food mechanically (by chewing) and chemically (by digestive juices that are produced throughout the system). The nutrients are then absorbed into the blood stream and carried around the body.

Food provides energy and nutrition, and a good diet can help people to stay healthy. Food is also important because eating is an enjoyable activity. Meals can be social occasions and provide structure in a person's day. Service users often look forward to them.

What happens

- Someone who has problems with their teeth, or whose false teeth don't fit very well, may find chewing difficult. They might dribble or develop sores at the corner of their mouth.

- If a service user's salivary glands (the glands in the mouth that produce saliva, or spit) are not working properly, they may have a dry mouth.

- Bad breath (halitosis) can be a sign of tooth decay or problems with the digestion.

- A service user's taste buds may stop working properly.

- A service user's ability to swallow can be affected by the position in which they are sitting or lying, or by muscle problems. Dysphagia is the medical term for difficulty with swallowing. Some people with dysphagia have problems swallowing certain food or liquids, while others cannot swallow at all.

- The glands that produce the digestive juices (enzymes) that digest food may not work properly.

- Wear and tear or disease could lead to problems with any part of a service user's digestive system. Their digestion might be slow or might not work very well.

- Constipation and/or diarrhoea can be caused by poor muscle tone and problems with absorbing food and liquid.

What this means for service users

- Service users may lose interest in food.

- If they don't eat enough, service users' energy levels may drop and their health may suffer.

- They may be afraid to eat certain foods because they think it will upset their stomach, or they might not drink enough liquid because they are worried about incontinence.

- They may become isolated because they are embarrassed about eating in front of other people.

What you can do

- Check service users' diets with the service users themselves or by checking their care plans.

- Encourage older people to eat little and often.

- If you are preparing food for service users, make sure it looks attractive and serve it in small, manageable portions.

- Only mince or mash food if absolutely necessary.

- If a service user is having trouble with their teeth, dentures or gums, talk to your supervisor so that an appointment can be arranged with a dentist.

- If a service user regularly dribbles or spills their food, make sure that their clothes are protected. Do so in a discreet way so that the person does not feel embarrassed or ashamed.

- If the service user is not interested in food, try offering them easy-to-eat foods such as custard, milk puddings, jelly or ice cream.

- Encourage a regular schedule for going to the toilet. This may prevent 'accidents' and therefore help to maintain a person's dignity, and it can help to reduce a service user's fear of incontinence.

- Make sure that the service user is cleaning their teeth or dentures regularly, or support them to do this.

- Make sure that drinks are always easily available. If a service user can't move around the home easily, leave a drink within their reach.

The respiratory and circulatory system

The lungs, heart and blood are all part of the respiratory and circulatory system. This is the system that provides our bodies with oxygen. When we breathe, oxygen from the air is absorbed into our bloodstream via our lungs, and the blood carries it to the rest of the body.

What happens

Lungs and trachea (windpipe). The tissues in a person's lungs can become diseased or their air passages can become blocked. This may be caused by the ageing process, by an infection or because the lungs have been damaged, perhaps by smoking or by working in a polluted environment. Fluid can accumulate on the lungs or the lung tissue can harden, which can cause breathing difficulties or a cough that won't go away.

Heart and blood vessels. As a person gets older, their heart and blood vessels (which carry the blood around the body) can become weaker and less elastic. The walls of the blood vessels can also become thicker because of a build-up of cholesterol – a fatty substance that occurs naturally in the body but that can be dangerous at high levels. These changes may cause a person's blood to flow slowly around the body or cause a blockage inside a blood vessel.

What this means for the service user

- A service user may find it difficult and tiring to breathe, and they may absorb less oxygen.

- Blockages in the blood vessels may stop oxygen getting to parts of a person's body. For example, a stroke is a blockage which prevents oxygen reaching brain cells, causing some brain cells to die.

- Poor circulation may also mean that not enough oxygen reaches a service user's skin or the tissue beneath – for example parts of the body that are under pressure from sitting or lying in one position, or the fingers or toes.

- A thrombosis, which is a blood clot that forms in a vein, can cause heart attacks, high blood pressure, swelling of the limbs, strokes or breathing difficulties.

What you can do

- Help the service user to sit in an upright position.

- Encourage the service user to open a window, even if for a short time, to allow some fresh air into the home.

- Encourage the person to do some gentle exercises to help their circulation. Arm raising/swinging exercises and deep breathing can be done from a sitting position.

- Offer to help the service user to blow or clean their nose.

- Read the chapter on first aid (*Chapter 7 – What to do in an emergency*) so that you know what to do in an emergency.

The urinary system and sex organs

Our kidneys regulate the amount of fluid in our bodies by removing excess water, salts and waste products from the blood. Urine from the kidneys is collected in the bladder and passed via the urethra.

What happens

- A person's kidneys may not function effectively because of an infection or disease.

- Minerals and other substances in a person's urine may collect over time and form what are known as kidney stones, which can be very painful.

- The muscles that people use when they go to the toilet may be damaged or work less effectively.

- Men may suffer from enlargement of the prostate gland – a gland below the bladder that contributes to the production of semen.

- Women may suffer from a dry, uncomfortable or itching vagina.

- Giving birth can weaken the muscles of the pelvic floor, which supports the bladder. This may mean some women are more likely to become incontinent as they get older.

Remember that in almost all cases, incontinence can be treated or strategies can be put in place to help avoid it. All service users who have incontinence problems should be assessed by a specialist professional (often known as a continence advisor).

What this means for the service user

- Problems with the urinary and sex organs can cause service users to feel embarrassed or ashamed. They might find it difficult to admit that they need help.

- They might become socially isolated if people are put off visiting their home because of unpleasant smells. Or the service user may avoid contact with other people because they are embarrassed about their incontinence.

- They may be in pain.

- Family tensions may arise, or a family carer may struggle to cope, because of the extra work associated with incontinence (such as additional laundry).

What you can do

- Make sure that all service users receive expert help and advice with continence issues.

- Strictly follow service users' care plans and toilet routines. Follow any instructions left by the continence adviser, community nurse or health visitor.

- If you notice that a service user's skin is being damaged because of incontinence, for example if you see red marks or soreness, make a note of this and report it to your supervisor.

- Encourage service users to wash frequently and to dry themselves carefully.

- Clean up any urine spilled on floors, and give lavatory and bedside mats a regular airing.

- Encourage or support service users to wash or clean their clothes regularly.

- Use perfumed air fresheners and talcum powder sparingly. They are only effective for a short period of time and may irritate a service user's nose, throat or lungs.

- Try to make sure that service users' homes are pleasant to visit, for example by letting some fresh air in to get rid of smells. Do this as tactfully as you can so that the service user doesn't feel offended or embarrassed.

- Service users may feel ashamed about incontinence or embarrassed about being helped to go to the toilet. Be sensitive to their feelings and carry out your role in a way that helps them to maintain their dignity. Your approach may differ depending on the individual.

The brain and nerves

The nervous system is the body's communication system. Electrical impulses pass to and from the brain and different parts of the body via a network of nerve cells, or neurons. These impulses carry messages from the body to the brain about sensations such as pressure, heat, cold and pain. The brain also sends out instructions to other parts of the body – for example to make our legs or arms move.

What happens

- There are a variety of conditions that can cause damage to the brain. These include strokes (sometimes called a cerebrovascular accident or CVA), disorders of the blood vessels of the brain or its covering membranes, or diseases such as Alzheimer's disease or Parkinson's disease, which damage the nerve cells in the brain. Tumours – whether they are cancerous or not – can cause pressure in the brain and stop it from working properly.

- Nerve fibres can be trapped.

- Nerve endings can be damaged which may stop them working or mean they work less effectively.

- The nerve covering (sheath) can be destroyed, interrupting the messages to and from the brain. This is what happens when someone has multiple sclerosis.

What this means for service users

- People who have diabetes may experience numbness (lack of feeling) in their feet and hands. This is called neuropathy. It may mean that a person can't sense pain or heat, which can lead to them injuring themselves or not seeking treatment for an injury.

- A service user's sense of touch may become less sensitive, so that they only feel strong sensations. Or they may be unusually sensitive, so that even gentle touch is painful. Their sense of touch might be distorted, for example they may feel a 'creeping' sensation on the skin when they are touched.

- A service user's muscles may be affected, making it difficult or impossible for them to move. If the muscles in their face are affected, they may dribble or have problems with eating.

- Memory may be affected, in particular short-term memory (see *Chapter 11 – Supporting people with dementia*).

- Damage to the nervous system may cause people to feel more tired.

- People may find it more difficult to communicate. They may have problems with speech and writing and be unable to interpret written words.

- A service user's hearing, sight or taste may be affected.

What you can do

- Understand that some of these conditions can be improved or cured. Ensure that any available help or treatment has been sought through your agency.

- Try to learn as much as possible about service users' health conditions and support them according to their individual needs. Ask your agency for further information.

- Check posture, diet and medication, especially if a service user is in pain.

- Encourage service users to think, talk and express opinions (see *Chapter 9 – Mental health*).

- Check service users' care plans, especially for personal and individual habits or routines they may have that may be associated with damage to the brain.

- Be careful not to tire out service users. Like everyone else, service users will have good days and bad days, and the level of activity they are capable of may vary from day to day.

- Note any change in service users' behaviour and report anything that causes you concern.

Sensory organs

The eye

Light passes through the eye's lens, which is situated behind the iris (the coloured part of the eye) and the pupil (the opening at the centre of the iris that allows light into the eye). The pupil gets larger or smaller to control the amount of light that enters the eye. When the light reaches the retina (a layer of light-sensitive cells at the back of the eye), the cells of the retina transmit information about what we are seeing to the brain.

The eye is protected by a membrane called the conjunctiva. Tears stop the eyes from drying out, and wash away dust and germs. The eyelids protect the eye and blinking keeps the surface of the eye moist.

What happens

- As a person gets older, the lens can thicken and cataracts can form – this is a cloudy layer that can make vision blurred or misty.

- The gland that produces tears, can produce too much or too little liquid. If a person doesn't produce enough tears, their eyes can become dry and 'scratchy'.

- The tear ducts drain away excess tears – if a person's tear ducts are blocked the fluid will stay in the eye rather than draining away.

- The eye may become infected or diseased, which can affect people's vision or cause them discomfort. Some examples are conjunctivitis (an infection of the conjunciva, the membrane that covers the eye) and glaucoma (when the pressure of fluid in the eye builds up).

What this means for the service user

- Cataracts can gradually get worse, affecting service users' sight and making reading, writing, moving about and recognising objects and people increasingly difficult. Cataracts can be removed with an operation; the person may have to wait until the cataracts have reached a certain thickness before they can have the operation.

- A person with glaucoma may lose their sight if the condition is not treated quickly.

- Some eye conditions lead to 'tunnel vision', which means a reduced field of vision – as though a person is wearing blinkers.

- Dry eyes can feel very uncomfortable.

- Even if they are registered blind, a blind or partially sighted person is likely to have some visual sensations. For example they may be able to detect darkness or brightness. They may need to wear dark glasses to protect their eyes. A partially sighted person may be able to see things under some conditions but not others.

- Service users who have problems with their vision will need to use extra concentration and energy to remember where things are, and this can be very tiring. If they need to learn their way around a new environment they may need extra time and support.

- Someone who used to be able to see may forget what things or colours are like, or have visual memories that are out of date.

- Blind or partially sighted service users who also have hearing problems are likely to have additional difficulty with communication and mobility.

What you can do

- Make sure a service user's spectacles are clean – whether or not they enable the service user to see.

- If the service user has tunnel vision, place objects within their field of vision.

- If a service user finds bright light uncomfortable, close or partially close the blinds or curtains, or suggest to the person that they move to a different position.

- Think about the home from the service user's point of view, and take care not to leave obstacles in their way. What might not seem to be an obstacle for you may cause problems for a service user.

- Be sure to leave items in their usual places, so the service user can find them more easily.

- If a service user has watering eyes, leave a box of tissues within their reach. Make a note and talk to your supervisor so that medical help can be sought if necessary.

- For service users with dry eyes, you could suggest helping them to use an eye bath, or talk to your supervisor as the person may benefit from a prescription of 'artificial tears'.

- Identify yourself when you arrive and let the person know when you are leaving.

- Speak to the service user clearly and naturally – there is no need to talk in a loud voice unless the person also has hearing difficulties. Use everyday language. For example it is fine to use words such as 'see' or 'look' in conversation.

- If you need to read instructions to the service user, do so clearly. If you leave a reminder or note for a person with partial sight, write it in large, bold letters.

The ear

Sound waves travel along a tube to a membrane (the ear drum) which vibrates. This moves the small bones in the middle ear, which pass the sound waves on to the inner ear. Here the sound waves make the 'cochlea', a fluid-filled tube, vibrate. Tiny cells in the cochlea pick up the vibrations and send them as nerve signals to the brain.

As well as enabling us to hear, the ears are important for our sense of balance, which can be affected by conditions of the ear.

What happens

- A person's ear drum may be punctured, which means it won't vibrate. The small bones of their middle ear may become fixed and unable to transmit the sound waves to the inner ear.

- The nerves that transmit information to the brain may be destroyed or damaged.

- Wax may accumulate in the tube of the outer ear.

- The outer or inner ear can become infected.

What this means for the service user

- Because hearing often gets worse slowly over time, and because of the association between hearing loss and old age, some service users may deny that they have hearing problems or try to hide it by guessing what people are saying to them.

- Hearing loss can make it much more difficult for the person to communicate and they may become lonely and isolated.

- A person with hearing loss may be able to hear very high or very low sounds, and they might find these sounds disturbing.

- As a person's hearing gets worse, they are likely to lose the ability to hear high notes before low notes. This means they might be able to hear man's voice better than a woman's.

- Hearing aids magnify sound but cannot pick out certain sounds, such as voices. They do not cure conditions of the ear which cause deafness.

- Wax in the ears may cause a service user to become temporarily deaf. This needs to be treated and may be a recurring problem.

- A person with tinnitus will hear a continual ringing, buzzing or humming sound in their ears that doesn't correspond with any external sound. This can disturb a person's concentration or sleep. A service user with tinnitus can become distressed or depressed.

- Infections in the ear can cause pain and loss of hearing. They should be treated as quickly as possible.

What you can do

- If a service user is in pain, report this to your supervisor straight away so that medical help can be arranged.

- Not many people are completely deaf, and it is important to make use of whatever hearing a service user has. Find out what they can hear, what they find helpful and whether there are any useful strategies you could learn to help you communicate with them and support them.

- Look directly at the service user when you speak to them so that they can see your mouth and lip read. Practise lip reading yourself.

- Say things clearly and a bit more slowly than usual.

- Be patient and prepared to say things more than once. If you have repeated something once or twice and the person still doesn't understand, try to say it using different words.

- Don't talk to a service user when you are behind them or while you are moving away from them.

- Talk in a slightly louder voice than usual, but do not shout. Shouting distorts the lip patterns, making lip reading more difficult, and you may come across as aggressive.

- Background noise can make it more difficult for a partially deaf person to hear you. Reduce other noises when you are talking to a deaf service user, for example by closing windows or temporarily turning off the radio or TV.

- Be prepared to describe sounds to remind service users what they are like.

- Use hand gestures, and, if a service user uses a communication system such as British Sign Language (BSL) or Makaton, try to learn some signs. Keep your hands away from your face while speaking, and speak at the same time as you sign.

- Adjust a person's hearing aid if it whistles – it may need to be turned down from full volume or it may whistle because the earpiece doesn't fit very well. If whistling is a constant problem, report this so that the person can get some specialist advice.

- Make sure service users are able to use their hearing aids. Learn how to help clean hearing aids. Remember to check whether the batteries need changing, and offer to help replace them (they are very small and can be difficult to handle). The NHS provides free batteries for NHS aids.

- Have a pencil and pad handy so that you can write down messages to each other.

- Knock loudly at the door.

- When phoning your client, let the telephone ring for longer than usual.

- Check the bell on the telephone is loud enough for the service user to hear. Fittings can be provided to make the telephone bell and the sound from the handset louder.

- Suggest a visit to the GP if you think a service user is becoming increasingly deaf, and discuss this with your supervisor.

- Suggest to a service user that they use earphones if playing their radio or television at high volume is causing a problem for their neighbours. They could also put on subtitles when watching the television.

The nose

The nose is an air passage that filters and moistens the air that we breathe in. The membrane covering the inside of the nose makes a sticky substance (mucus) which traps small particles. At the back of the nose cavities are the nerves that enable us to detect smells. The sense of smell plays a part in our sense of taste.

What happens

- An infection may cause a person to produce extra mucus (nasal catarrh), which may block the nose.

- Drugs may affect the sense of smell.

- Some conditions or a head injury may damage or destroy the nerves that carry the sense of smell.

- Small growths (polyps) may develop in the nasal passages.

What this means to the service user

- The service user may be at risk because they can't smell signs of danger, such as gas or bad food.

- Food may taste bland to a person who has lost their sense of smell and they may lose their appetite.

- The service user may be unaware of bad smells in the home, such as urine, pet smells or cigarette smoke. Unpleasant smells may put people off visiting, and the service user may become lonely and isolated as a result.

What you can do

- Check that food stored in the person's home is fresh. If not, suggest to the service user that they throw it away.

- Remind the service user of what to do in emergency situations, such as a fire or gas leak.

- Try to deal with the causes of unpleasant smells.

- Try to find ways of encouraging the service user to eat – see 'The tongue' below.

The tongue

Our tongue helps us to move food around in our mouths when we chew, to taste our food and to form words when we speak. There are many nerve endings in the tongue, which means it also has a highly developed sense of touch. Everyone has taste buds on their throat and palate as well as on their tongue.

What happens

- Drugs can affect the way taste buds function.

- Inflammation of the mouth or gums, or ulcers or tumours may cause discomfort and affect people's sense of taste.

What this means for the service user

- Food may seem tasteless, which may mean that a service user will lose their appetite and lose weight.

- Service users may use more pepper, salt or other seasonings to make their food more flavoursome.

What you can do

- Find out if a service user's sense of taste is affected, and whether there are particular foods that taste unpleasant to them.

- If a service user has lost their sense of taste, encourage meals with different textures to make up for the lack of taste.

- Observe and note the state of a service user's mouth, especially if they have halitosis (bad breath), and discuss further action with your supervisor.

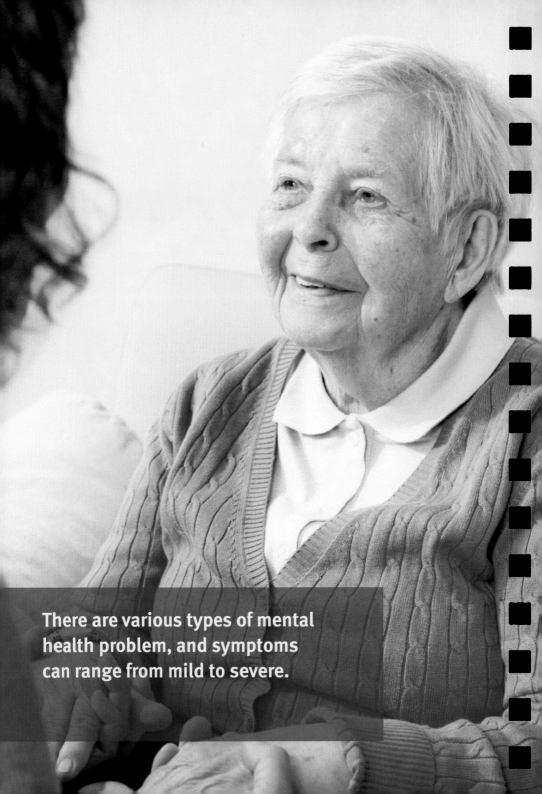

There are various types of mental
health problem, and symptoms
can range from mild to severe.

9 Mental health

Mental health problems are more common than you might think – one in four people will experience a mental health problem in any given year. While your role may be to support service users' physical or practical needs, it is also important to be aware of their emotional and mental wellbeing.

There are various types of mental health problem, and symptoms can range from mild to severe. Mental health problems can be treated, often with talking therapies, medication or a combination of the two, and many people recover from mental illness, or keep their symptoms under control.

This chapter gives basic details about some of the most common types of mental health problem. It also provides information about mental capacity and how it applies to your work.

If you are concerned that a service user is having problems with their mental health, talk to your supervisor.

Depression

Every now and again, most of us feel sad or 'low', or lose our motivation to do things. However, if these feelings last for more than two weeks, or come back repeatedly, and begin to affect a person's life, it could mean that they have depression. Some people will become depressed for no obvious reason, while for others it may be triggered by a significant change in their life. The death of a loved one, the onset of a long-term illness, loneliness or a loss of independence are all possible causes of depression. Depression is thought to affect one in six people at some point in their lives.

A service user who is depressed might:

- Feel sad, low-spirited, hopeless, empty or without emotion for much of the time every day.

- Feel tired and lack energy, doing less and less.

- Feel irritable or impatient or prone to crying.

- Find it hard to concentrate and make decisions, or be preoccupied.

- Get no pleasure out of life, or from things that they usually enjoy.

- Be preoccupied by negative thoughts, lack confidence or self-esteem.

- Wake up early, have difficulty sleeping or sleep more.

- Not eat properly, either losing or putting on weight.

- Use more tobacco, alcohol or drugs than usual.

- Distance themselves from others, not asking for help.

- Neglect their appearance or surroundings.

- In extreme cases, attempt self-harm (e.g. cutting arms) or suicide.

You can help by:

- Acknowledging the service user's feelings. Take the person seriously, don't try to jolly them along and don't tell them to 'cheer up' or 'snap out of it'.

- Allowing time for listening.

- Encouraging the service user to discuss how they feel with their family doctor (GP).

- Suggesting something practical for the service user to do, for example write a letter or make a phone call.

- Encouraging the service user to look ahead by doing something practical and helping them with a plan of action – remember to follow this up on your next visit.

- Encouraging the service user to have some social contact and reporting any concerns you have to your supervisor.

- Providing gentle encouragement to maintain their personal care.

- Identifying activities or conversation that still provides pleasure.

- Being on the alert for people whose depression is increasing and discussing your concerns with your supervisor, particularly if the service user is expressing thoughts about harming themselves or ending their life.

Anxiety

We all get anxious in certain situations, but extreme anxiety can have a negative affect on someone's everyday life. Anxiety has physical effects, caused by the release of the hormone adrenalin into the body. These include high blood pressure, tension in the muscles, rapid breathing and feeling sick. Anxiety also affects a person's mental wellbeing. It can be treated in various ways, including drugs and talking therapies. Learning relaxation techniques or making lifestyle changes can also help people to cope better with anxiety.

A service user who is anxious might:

- Feel fearful, irritable or tearful.

- Find it difficult to concentrate or relax.

- Have trouble sleeping.

- Become depressed.

- Find it difficult to enjoy leisure time.

- Drink alcohol or take drugs to try and cope with their feelings.

- Have panic attacks, which are sudden episodes of extreme anxiety. A person having a panic attack might experience a pounding heart, chest pains, shaky limbs, nausea, and a feeling of being out of control. These episodes can be very frightening and distressing.

Anxiety can also take other forms, including:

- Phobias, where a person becomes anxious because of an irrational fear, such as a fear of spiders, crowded places or going outside.

- Obsessive compulsive disorder (OCD). A person with OCD may think unwanted thoughts over and over again, and/or feel compelled to carry out a particular activity repeatedly. For example, they may constantly think about being covered in germs and feel the need to repeatedly wash their hands.

- Post-traumatic stress disorder, which can develop after a person has seen or been involved in an extremely distressing or stressful event, such as a serious accident, physical attack or violent death.

You can help by:

- Listening and taking the service user's feelings seriously.

- Talking through what you are doing and trying to create agreed sequences of actions, without repetitions.

- Encouraging a good diet and regular meals.

- Reporting any concerns you have about the service user to your agency and finding out whether they have been offered any professional help.

Schizophrenia

There is some uncertainty about the nature of schizophrenia; some experts believe it involves a range of different disorders that share similar symptoms. The symptoms can be managed with medication and psychological treatment. Some people recover completely, while others may have occasional episodes of illness or live with the symptoms throughout their lives.

Schizophrenia is often misunderstood. Two commonly held myths about people with schizophrenia are that they have a 'split personality' or are likely to be violent. In fact, incidences of someone with schizophrenia committing acts of violence are very rare.

A service user who has schizophrenia might:

- Have jumbled or confused thoughts, which may not make sense to others.

- See things, hear voices or smell things that other people can't see, hear or smell. These are called hallucinations.

- Have distressing beliefs or experiences that are not based on reality – for example, they might believe they are being followed or watched, or that their thoughts are being controlled by an external force or person. These are called delusions.

- Become disorganised, unpredictable or agitated.

- Neglect their appearance or personal hygiene.

- Withdraw from other people.

You can help by:

- Monitoring the service user's mental wellbeing and reporting any changes in their behaviour to your supervisor.

- Letting your supervisor know if the service user is not taking prescribed medication.

- Being patient and not getting angry about any unusual or antisocial behaviour.

- Acknowledging what the service user is experiencing. Be honest, but don't deny or contradict the person's experience – they may find this alienating or upsetting. You could say, for example, "I accept that you can hear a voice, but I can't hear it." It can be more helpful to focus on the way the service user is feeling rather than what they are experiencing.

- Helping the service user to eat well and, if possible, encouraging regular sleeping patterns.

Bipolar disorder (previously called manic depression)

Bipolar disorder causes extreme mood swings. A person with the illness will have periods when they are highly active, excited and happy (this is known as mania). They will also have periods when they feel extremely low and depressed. Some people only experience a few of these episodes during a lifetime, while others have regular 'highs' and 'lows'. This pattern can interfere with everyday life and relationships. The symptoms of bipolar disorder can be treated with drugs, and some people find talking therapies helpful. People with the illness can learn to recognise when they are about to go into a high or low phase, which means they can get help to manage the symptoms.

A service user having a 'manic' episode might:

- Be full of energy and talk very quickly.

- Be over optimistic or euphoric (excessively 'high').

- Be unusually impatient or get annoyed easily.

- Make irrational or ill-judged decisions, for example they might spend lots of money on something they can't afford.

- Talk about grand plans.

- Have an increased interest in sex.

- Sleep or eat less than usual.

- Behave in a way that is out of character, or do things that seem risky or that could be harmful.

- Have illogical thoughts, delusional beliefs or hallucinations.

During a 'depressive' (low) episode they might:

- Feel a lack of hope, despairing or empty.

- Lose interest in day-to-day life.

- Feel exhausted and have problems with their sleep patterns.

- Have suicidal thoughts.

You can help by:

- Maintaining a consistent manner rather than reflecting the service user's mood.

- Acknowledging that the service user's experiences and feelings are real for them. However, it is important not to collude with any unrealistic plans or ideas.

- Involving the service user in the practical activities of your tasks.

- Not showing any impatience or irritation that you might feel.

- Reporting any concerns about the service user to your supervisor.

Mental Capacity

The expression "mental capacity" means the ability to make decisions for yourself. It is an important area to be familiar with, as you may meet service users who struggle to make some decisions for themselves, and you may then become the 'decision maker' on their behalf.

There is legislation in England, Wales and Scotland that provides guidance on the issues of mental capacity and decision making, to people who provide care to service users.

The Mental Capacity Act (England and Wales) 2005 and the Adults with Incapacity (Scotland) Act 2000 are laws that support and protect people who are unable to make decisions for themselves. Someone might be unable to make decisions because of a mental health problem, a brain injury, learning difficulties or an illness such as dementia. The legislation assumes that everyone has mental capacity unless it is proven otherwise.

The aim of the Acts is to enable people to make as many decisions as they can. It allows people to make decisions about future medical treatment before they lose their mental capacity (their ability to make decisions), and to appoint someone else to make decisions about their health, welfare and finances when they can no longer do so themselves. The Acts also enable decisions to be made by others in a person's best interests, if they are unable to do so and have not indicated their choices in advance.

The Mental Capacity (Health, Welfare and Finance) Bill is currently under discussion in Northern Ireland but the principles discussed here about mental capacity still apply to those providing care in Northern Ireland.

Information regarding mental capacity

Whether a service user might need support in making decisions should be recorded during the process of agreeing their care plan. If they might need support then the care plan should contain:

- A record of any prior wishes or beliefs that may help decisions to be made in the service user's best interests.

- Information about family, friends or advocates who may be consulted about the service user's choices and preferences, as well as guidance on the circumstances in which they might be consulted.

- Details of anyone who has been officially appointed to act on the service user's behalf (for example an Attorney or Court Deputy).

- Information about whether the service user has made an advance decision, for example about future medical treatment.

Mental capacity and your role

Make yourself familiar with the principles of the relevant Acts and the content of your agency's policies and procedures in relation to them.

In your day-to-day work it is important to remember the following:

- All service users have a right to make their own decisions and are assumed to have mental capacity unless proved otherwise.

- Don't make assumptions about whether the service user has the capacity to understand and make a decision about something – check!

- A service user's ability to make a decision can be affected by the time of day or the effects of medication, for example. If possible, wait until a time when the service user is most able to make the decision.

- If a service user doesn't have the capacity to make complicated decisions, don't assume that they can't make any decisions.

- There will be times when you will need to make a decision on behalf of a service user. The decisions you make must be in the best interests of the service user and maintain their rights and freedoms.

- Check the service user's care plan for any information relating to decision making.

- If you make a decision on a service user's behalf, follow your agency's guidance for recording the steps you took to assess the service user's capacity.

- Use your knowledge of the service user when you are considering a decision. Think about what they might choose, based on what you know about their culture, background and preferences.

Talk to your supervisor if:

- You believe that a service user's ability to make decisions is changing. If necessary, a reassessment of the service user's mental capacity can be arranged.

- You have any queries about the laws about mental capacity in your part of the UK, or the situations in which you should make decisions for a service user and the types of decisions you can make on their behalf.

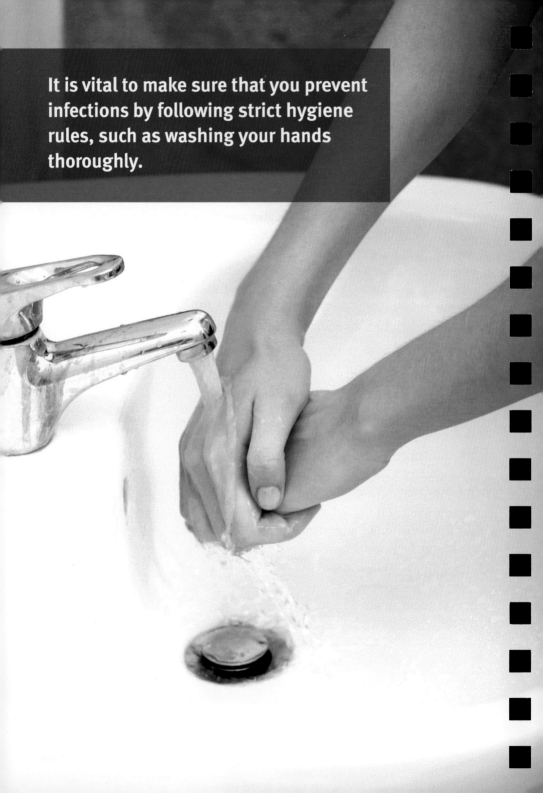

It is vital to make sure that you prevent infections by following strict hygiene rules, such as washing your hands thoroughly.

10   Common health conditions

In this chapter you'll find brief information about some of the health conditions that you are likely to come across during your work. To help understand how best to support your service user with their condition you can:

• Ask the service user

• Talk to the service user's family members or carers

• Refer to the service user's care plan

• Look in general guides and books written for careworkers

• Seek help and information from charities that support people with particular conditions

• Ask your supervisor for more training

Infections

An infection is the invasion of the body by disease-causing organisms such as bacteria or viruses. Infections can be passed on by close contact with another person (for example, cold sores), through water (cholera), air (the common cold), food (such as salmonella in undercooked chicken), or insects (such as malaria from a mosquito bite).

Common symptoms of infection could be redness, swelling, heat, pain and a loss of function in the affected area. It can also cause a high temperature, weakness, loss of appetite and feeling unwell. The immune system may get weaker as a person gets older, and can also be affected by certain medication or hospital treatment.

The infections that most commonly affect older people are chest or urinary infections, both of which cause people to feel unwell and possibly feverish and confused. A person with a urinary infection is likely to have dark-coloured urine that smells unpleasant. Another common infection among older people is cellulitis, which can occur when ulcers and wounds become infected. In all these cases you should talk to your agency to make sure the person gets medical help straight away.

If a service user has an infection, ensure that:

- They drink plenty of fluids so that they don't become dehydrated

- You change their clothes or the temperature of the room to reduce a high temperature

- They are comfortable

- They get plenty of rest

- They get medical advice

It is also vital to make sure that you prevent infections (see *Chapter 5 – Health and safety at work*) by following strict hygiene rules, such as:

- Washing your hands thoroughly

- Wearing disposable gloves and aprons

- Covering the mouth and nose with a tissue when sneezing or coughing

- Covering any cuts or grazes

- Disposing of waste properly

Conditions that might affect service users

Anaemia

Anaemia is a condition where the amount of haemoglobin in the blood is below the normal level, or there are fewer red blood cells than normal. There are several different types of anaemia and each one has a different cause, although iron deficiency anaemia is the most common type. Other forms of anaemia can be caused by a lack of vitamin B12 or folic acid in the body.

Arthritis

Arthritis is a common condition that causes pain and inflammation within a joint. There are many different types of arthritis that cause a wide range of symptoms. Two of the most common are osteoarthritis and rheumatoid arthritis. There are many different symptoms of arthritis and the symptoms you experience will vary depending on the type of arthritis you have. However, common arthritic symptoms include:

- Joint pain, tenderness and stiffness

- Inflammation in and around the joints

- Restricted movement of the joints, which may affect walking, movement and grip.

- Warmth and redness of the skin over the affected joint

- Weakness and muscle wasting (loss of muscle strength and size)

Asthma

Asthma is a common long-term condition that can cause a cough, wheezing and breathlessness. Asthma is caused by inflammation of the airways. When someone comes into contact with something that irritates their lungs, known as a trigger, their airways become narrow, the muscles around them tighten and there is an increase in the production of sticky mucus (phlegm). This leads to symptoms including:

- Difficulty breathing
- Wheezing and coughing
- A tight chest

Asthma is most often treated with drugs to make breathing easier and reduce inflammation.

A severe onset of symptoms is known as an asthma attack or an 'acute asthma exacerbation'. Asthma attacks may require hospital treatment and can sometimes be life-threatening, although this is rare.

Bronchitis

Bronchitis is an infection of the main airways of the lungs (bronchi), which causes them to become irritated and inflamed. The main symptom is a cough which may bring up yellow-grey mucus. Bronchitis may also cause a sore throat, wheezing and a blocked nose.

Cancer

Cancer is a disease caused by normal cells changing so that they grow in an uncontrolled way. The uncontrolled growth causes a lump to form, called a tumour. If not treated, the tumour can cause problems in one or more of the following ways:

- Spreading into normal tissues nearby

- Causing pressure or obstruction to other organs

- Spreading to other parts of the body through the lymphatic system or bloodstream

- Causing rupture of blood vessels inside the body

Cerebral Palsy

Cerebral palsy is a general term covering a number of neurological conditions that affect a person's movement and coordination. Neurological conditions affect the brain and nervous system. Cerebral palsy is caused by damage to the brain, which normally occurs before, during or soon after birth.

People with cerebral palsy tend to have problems with their muscle tone (the unconscious ability to contract or relax muscles as needed) such as:

- Hypertonia: increased muscle tone, which can make them appear stiff or rigid

- Hypotonia: decreased muscle tone, which makes them appear floppy

People with cerebral palsy also tend to favour one side of the body over the other, which can make their posture appear unusual.

Cystic Fibrosis

Cystic fibrosis is a genetic condition in which the lungs and digestive system become clogged with thick sticky mucus. Symptoms usually start in early childhood and include:

- Persistent cough
- Repeated chest infections
- Poor weight gain and prolonged diarrhoea

There is no cure for cystic fibrosis. So the aim of treatment is to ease the symptoms and make the condition easier to live with.

Dementia

Dementia is a syndrome (a group of related symptoms) that is associated with an ongoing decline of the brain and its abilities. These include:

- Memory
- Thinking
- Language
- Understanding
- Judgement

People with dementia may also become apathetic, or have problems controlling their emotions or behaving appropriately in social situations. Aspects of their personality may change, or they may see or hear things that other people do not, or they may have false beliefs. Most cases of dementia are caused by damage to the structure of the brain. Usually dementia occurs in people who are 65 or over. The older you get, the more likely you are to develop it. Dementia is slightly more common in women than in men.

Different types of dementia:

- Alzheimer's disease, where small clumps of protein, known as plaques, begin to develop around brain cells. This disrupts the normal workings of the brain.

- Vascular dementia, where problems with blood circulation result in parts of the brain not receiving enough blood and oxygen.

- Dementia with Lewy bodies, where abnormal structures, known as Lewy bodies, develop inside the brain.

- Frontotemporal dementia, where the frontal and temporal lobes (two parts of the brain) begin to shrink. Unlike other types of dementia, frontotemporal dementia usually develops in people who are under 65. It is much rarer than other types of dementia.

See *Chapter 11 – Supporting people with dementia*, for more information.

Diabetes

Diabetes is a long-term condition caused by too much glucose (sugar) in the blood.

The two main types of diabetes are:

- Type 1 diabetes – the body's immune system attacks and destroys the cells that produce insulin. As no insulin is produced, glucose levels increase, which can seriously damage the body's organs.

- Type 2 diabetes – the body does not produce enough insulin, or the body's cells do not react to insulin. (This is known as insulin resistance).

The main symptoms of diabetes are:

- Feeling very thirsty
- Urinating frequently, particularly at night
- Feeling very tired
- Weight loss and loss of muscle bulk

There are a number of treatments for diabetes, mainly eating a low-carbohydrate diet, medication to improve insulin absorption, or insulin injections.

Dysphasia

Dysphasia can be caused by a head injury, loss of blood supply to the brain (for example, during a stroke), infection or inflammation of the brain, or brain tumour. People with dysphasia may have problems in communicating what they are thinking, with their ability to talk and write being impaired. They may also have problems understanding what is said to them.

Epilepsy

Epilepsy is a condition that affects the brain and causes repeated seizures, also known as fits. The severity of the seizures can differ from person to person. Some people simply experience a 'trance-like' state for a few seconds or minutes, while others lose consciousness and have convulsions (uncontrollable shaking of the body).

Gangrene

Gangrene is a serious condition in which a loss of blood supply causes tissue to die. It can affect any part of the body but typically starts in the toes, feet, fingers and hands (the extremities). Gangrene can occur as a result of an injury, infection or a long-term condition that affects blood circulation. Symptoms of gangrene include: the affected area of tissue changes colour, such as turning red to brown to black; a loss of sensation in the affected area, or the area of tissue becomes extremely painful; the affected tissue develops black blisters and begins producing a foul-smelling pus. Gangrene can develop quickly as a result of some diseases and requires urgent treatment. If you see any of these symptons, contact your supervisor immediately.

Heart Disease

Heart disease is the term that describes what happens when your heart's blood supply is blocked or interrupted by a build-up of fatty substances in the coronary arteries. Heart disease can lead to complex problems such as angina, heart attack or heart failure (see below).

Angina – This can begin as a mild, uncomfortable feeling that is similar to indigestion. However, a severe angina attack can cause a feeling of heaviness or tightness, usually in the centre of the chest, which may spread to the arms, neck, jaw, back or stomach. Angina is often triggered by physical activity or stressful situations. The symptoms usually pass in less than 10 minutes and can be relieved by resting or prescribed medication. Angina which does not respond to treatment may be serious and you should call the emergency services if the service user is in pain or distress.

Heart attack (Myocardial infarction) – a serious medical emergency in which the supply of blood to the heart is suddenly blocked, usually by a blood clot. Lack of blood to the heart can seriously damage the heart muscle. Symptoms can include:

- Chest pain: the chest can feel like it is being squeezed or compressed by a heavy object, and pain can radiate from the chest to the jaw, neck, arms and back

- Shortness of breath

- Feeling weak and/or lightheaded

- Overwhelming feeling of anxiety

It is important to stress that not everyone experiences severe chest pain; often the pain can be mild and mistaken for indigestion.

Heart failure – a serious condition where the heart has difficulty pumping enough blood around the body. It usually occurs because the heart muscle has become too weak or stiff to work properly. If you have heart failure it does not mean that your heart is about to stop working. Breathlessness, feeling very tired, and swollen legs, ankles and feet are the main symptoms of heart failure. Sometimes, the symptoms of heart failure can develop quickly (acute heart failure). However, they usually develop gradually, over time (chronic heart failure).

HIV and AIDS

HIV stands for human immunodeficiency virus. The virus attacks the immune system, and weakens your ability to fight infections and disease. HIV is found in the body fluids of an infected person, which includes semen and vaginal fluids, blood, breast milk, and inside the anus. AIDS is the final stage of HIV infection, when your body can no longer fight life-threatening infections. There is no cure for HIV, but there are treatments to enable most people with the virus to live a long and healthy life.

Hypothermia

Hypothermia happens when a person's body temperature drops below 35°C (95°F). Normal body temperature is around 37°C (98.6°F). Hypothermia can quickly become life-threatening and should be treated as a medical emergency. Hypothermia is usually caused by being in a cold environment. It can be triggered by a combination of things, including being exposed to the cold for a long time – this can be outdoors in cold conditions, in a poorly heated room or being in cold water. Mild symptoms include shivering, tiredness and confusion. But as the temperature drops, shivering becomes more violent and a person is likely to become delirious, struggle to breathe and may become unconscious.

Motor Neurone Disease

Motor neurone disease is a rare condition that progressively damages the nervous system, causing the muscles to waste away. It occurs when specialist nerve cells, called motor neurones, stop working properly. In its early stages, motor neurone disease causes symptoms such as: a weakened grip, which can cause difficulty picking up or holding objects; a general feeling of tiredness; muscle pains and cramps. As the damage progresses, the symptoms become more debilitating. In the final stages of the disease, a person with the condition will be unable to move their body, talk or eat, and their breathing difficulties will worsen.

Multiple Sclerosis

Multiple sclerosis (MS) is a disease affecting nerves in the brain and spinal cord, causing problems with muscle movement, balance and vision. Each nerve fibre in the brain and spinal cord is surrounded by a layer of protein called myelin, which protects the nerve and helps electrical signals from the brain travel to the rest of the body. In MS, the myelin becomes damaged. This disrupts the transfer of these nerve signals, causing a wide range of potential symptoms, such as:

- Vision problems
- Balance problems
- Dizziness
- Muscle stiffness and uncontrolled muscle movements (spasm)
- Difficulties with balance and co-ordination
- Feeling very tired during the day
- Bladder problems

Parkinson's Disease

Parkinson's disease is a condition in which part of the brain becomes progressively more damaged over many years (a progressive neurological condition). The three main symptoms of Parkinson's disease are related to movement:

- Involuntary shaking of particular parts of the body – known as tremor

- Physical movements become very slow – known as bradykinesia

- Muscle stiffness that can make everyday tasks such as getting out of a chair very difficult – this is known as rigidity

A person with Parkinson's disease can also experience a wide range of symptoms unrelated to movement (non-motor symptoms) such as depression, daytime sleepiness and dysphagia (difficulties swallowing).

Pneumonia

Pneumonia is inflammation (swelling) of the tissue in one or both of the lungs. It is usually caused by an infection. At the end of the breathing tubes in the lungs are clusters of tiny air sacs. In pneumonia, these tiny sacs become inflamed and fill up with fluid. Common symptoms of pneumonia include:

- Difficulty breathing
- Coughing
- Fever

Stroke ("Cerebrovascular Accident" or "CVA")

A stroke is a serious medical condition that occurs when the blood supply to part of the brain is cut off. The main symptoms of stroke can be remembered with the word **FAST:** Face-Arms-Speech-Time.

- **F**ace – Has their face fallen on one side? Can they smile?

- **A**rms – Can they raise both arms and keep them there?

- **S**peech – Is their speech slurred?

- **T**ime – Time to call 999 for emergency help if you see any single one of these signs.

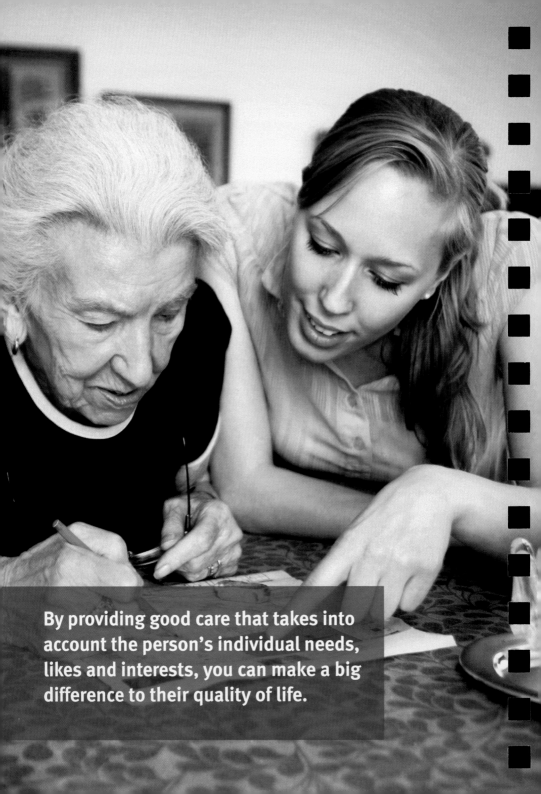

By providing good care that takes into account the person's individual needs, likes and interests, you can make a big difference to their quality of life.

11   Supporting people with dementia

Around two-thirds of people who have dementia live at home, so it is likely that some of your service users will be people with dementia.

Caring for a person with dementia can be challenging but it can also be very satisfying. By providing good care that takes into account the person's individual needs, likes and interests, you can make a big difference to their quality of life. It helps if you can take a flexible approach to your work; you'll also need to show plenty of understanding, patience and good humour.

This chapter gives a brief introduction to dementia and how you can best support people living with the illness. Find out more by going on specialist training or by talking to your supervisor or to a community mental health nurse.

About dementia

Dementia is a term used to describe a range of conditions that damage cells in the brain. The most common form of dementia is Alzheimer's disease. Other types include vascular dementia (caused by strokes in the brain), dementia with Lewy bodies and frontotemporal dementia. Dementia is a progressive disease, which means the symptoms get worse over time.

There is no cure for dementia, but drug treatments and coping strategies can help slow down the progress of the disease or help to manage the symptoms.

Dementia is most likely to affect older people, although significant numbers of people under the age of 65 develop dementia.

Signs of dementia

Different types of dementia have slightly different symptoms, but they usually include confusion, memory problems and the loss of everyday skills.

A person with dementia might:

- Have trouble remembering things that happened a short time ago. This might mean they ask the same question several times or carry out the same task repeatedly. (However, people with dementia can often remember things that happened many years ago.)

- Lose their way on a journey that they have done many times before.

- Feel confused, even in a familiar environment.

- Find it hard to follow the thread of a conversation or struggle to find the right words.

- Do things that seem unusual, like putting their reading glasses in the fridge or wanting to go out for a walk late at night.

- Behave in a way that is unusual for them – for example a person who used to be calm might become aggressive or rude.

- Become suspicious that people are stealing from them.

- Seem to be living in the past, for example they might insist that it is time to go to work even though they retired years ago.

As a person's dementia gets worse, they might lose the ability to recognise friends and family or carry out day-to-day tasks such as cooking or getting dressed. In the later stages of the disease mobility, communication, continence, eating and drinking can all be severely affected, resulting in the person becoming more dependent on carers.

If you work with a service user who already has a diagnosis of dementia – it is very important to monitor and report any changes in abilities, to ensure that care and support can be changed accordingly.

If a service user begins to show signs of dementia – make a note of this and let your line manager know, so that the person can be assessed. An early diagnosis is important, as it will mean that the person can access a range of information, advice, treatment and additional support if they need it.

Make sure you don't confuse dysphasia (difficulty with speech and language) with dementia. A service user with dysphasia may say things that seem confused but this is because they have difficulty with communication rather than their internal thought process. (See *Chapter 10 – Common health conditions*)

Getting to know the person with dementia

It is important to see beyond the symptoms of dementia and recognise that people with dementia are individuals. Find out as much as you can about a service user who has dementia by talking to the person themselves or their family and friends. Knowing more about their life history, culture and religion and current preferences will:

- Help you to provide care in a way that makes the service user feel comfortable.

- Provide clues that may help you to deal with any unusual behaviour.

- Give you things to talk about, which will make your visits more enjoyable for both of you and help you to build a good relationship.

Supporting service users who have dementia

Helping with tasks

By enabling them to do as much as possible for themselves, you will help service users with dementia to maintain their sense of self-worth.

- Break down tasks into small stages so that the service user can get involved in some of the stages, even if they can't do the whole task by themselves.

- As far as possible, help service users to make their own decisions. They might find lots of options confusing, so you could try suggesting one thing at a time. See *Chapter 9 – Mental health,* for more information about mental capacity and decision making.

- Try talking to the person about what you are doing, as this can be reassuring and help the service user to focus on the task. For example, when washing someone, you could talk about the scent of the soap, and offer it for the person to smell and so on.

- A person with dementia might be able to do more on some days than on others. Adapt your approach to tasks and the way you communicate with the person accordingly.

- Note how any special aids are used, such as a compliance aid for drugs. Talk to your manager about other aids or adaptations to the home if you think they could help a service user to continue to live independently.

- Check that you understand what drugs the person should be taking if this forms part of your role, and report back any mishap or problem.

- Don't worry too much about sticking to 'normality' as long as the service user is safe and comfortable. For example, it probably doesn't matter if they choose to eat an unusual combination of foods as long as they are getting enough to eat.

- Your time will be limited, but try not to rush through tasks as this can be distressing for the person with dementia. If you find that you don't have enough time for your tasks because the person's dementia is getting worse, discuss this with your supervisor.

Communication

- Introduce yourself to the person with dementia and explain you are there to help them if they are unsure who you are.

- It might be difficult to understand a service user who has dementia, or to know whether they have understood you. Be patient and allow the person time to find the right words or to process information. Using their name frequently can help maintain concentration and focus.

- People with dementia may need regular prompts and reminders to complete their daily activity. Be prepared to find different ways to say the same thing and keep your tone of voice friendly.

- Drop down to a person's eye level when you talk to them. Don't stand over them or stand too close to them, as this can seem intimidating.

- People with dementia may enjoy talking about earlier periods in their life, so encourage this. As well as bringing them enjoyment it will help you to establish a good working relationship.

- If a service user has lost their language skills, their body language and facial expression can give you clues about how they are feeling.

- Notes can act as useful reminders. Be inventive – for example you could draw a clock face to show the time.

Dealing with challenging or unusual behaviour

Dementia can cause a person to behave in ways that are out of character. They may be aggressive (physically or verbally), shout or scream, behave in sexually inappropriate ways or constantly repeat certain phrases or actions. These types of behaviour may be caused by changes in the person's brain, or they could be a reaction to feelings of frustration, anxiety or distress.

- Think about whether repeated actions relate to something in the person's past, such as their job. If so, you could use this as a topic for conversation. Constant repetition of the same actions could also signal that the person is bored and needs more stimulation.

- Someone who constantly calls out may be seeing something that isn't really there (a hallucination) or they may be in pain.

- If a service user wants to do something that seems unusual, such as going for a walk late at night, you could try to engage them in another activity or distract them by starting a conversation. However, you could enable the person to do what they want to do, even if it seems odd to you, if it avoids distress and if there is no risk to their welfare.

- Remember that it is the dementia that is causing the person to behave in a challenging way. Don't take it personally if they are aggressive or rude towards you. Avoid getting angry or 'punishing' the person in any way.

- Dealing with this type of behaviour is not easy. Find time between visits to acknowledge your frustrations and to plan helpful strategies for future visits, so that you don't carry negativity with you. Talk to your supervisor or colleagues to share experiences and tips.

- People with dementia may forget the usual social rules or behave in a sexually inappropriate way – for example taking off their clothes. Respond calmly and do all you can to maintain their dignity, particularly if they are in a public place.

- Listen to advice from the service user's family members; they may have already identified the causes or triggers for a person's behaviour and suggest helpful ways of dealing with it.

- Try to identify any triggers for aggressive behaviour. For example, does the person tend to become stressed if there is lots of noise and bustle, if they feel rushed or if they think their privacy is under threat? If you can identify triggers this will help you to take steps to avoid or minimise these situations.

- If a service user becomes aggressive, try to keep calm and give them lots of space. If you are worried about your own safety, leave the room (or the house) and contact your supervisor straight away to let them know. If you know that someone has been physically violent before, think about your position when you are in a room with them and make sure you can leave easily if you need to.

Maintaining nutrition and hydration

People with advanced dementia may need particular help with eating, drinking and remembering to take medication.

- Meals and drinks should be placed within easy reach and where they can be seen.

- It may be necessary to prompt people to eat and drink repeatedly during a meal, reminding and encouraging them to eat enough to meet their needs.

- Food and drinks should not just be left in a room for a person with dementia to eat by themselves, unless you are absolutely sure you can expect them to do so.

- It is important to check that food has been eaten. Do not assume that food and drink left uneaten was just because the person wasn't hungry.

- It may be necessary to note down in the service user's care records how much they ate. Some people may have a special chart in their records for this. Missed and partially eaten meals should also be recorded.

- If there is concern that meals are not being eaten, or that not enough drinks are being taken during the day you should inform your supervisor and members of the family.

- If you have insufficient time to assist the person with their meal or taking drinks, you should inform your supervisor so that more time can be made available.

Managing medication

- Unless you are sure that a person with dementia can remember to take their medicines, you should NOT leave medication out for them.

- Some people with dementia may take the wrong medication or too much medication without realising it. If supplies of medication are to be kept out of reach, this should be discussed with the person, their family carers and your supervisor and this should clearly be explained in the care plan.

- Unless the care plan suggests otherwise you should stay with the person while they take their medication. Check that the medications have all been taken before recording this on their medication administration record sheet (MAR).

- If you find that previous medication has not been taken, or the person refuses to take medicines that are due to them, record this in their records. Talk to your supervisor if there is any doubt that medicines are not being taken.

- It is generally not acceptable to hide medicines in food, or to crush tablets to make them easier to take. In rare situations that this has been agreed, you must follow the directions in the care plan and medicine chart carefully.

Maintaining dignity

As with all service users, a person with dementia needs to be valued and respected as an individual and their self-esteem and dignity maintained.

- Dementia can be a socially isolating condition. You must always include a person in conversation, even if it is difficult for them to join in. You must always treat people with dementia as a valued person and avoid talking over them, or ignoring what is known about their wishes or preferences, even if they cannot express them.

- When helping a person with dementia with intimate tasks, use the techniques that you would use with any other service user to maintain their dignity and privacy.

- A person who has dementia may see the world differently, and may say things that are not true. Or they may make mistakes or get very simple tasks wrong. In this case, respond in a sensitive way so that you don't make the person feel foolish.

- Laughter can relieve the tension in a difficult situation, but always make sure you are laughing with the person and not at them.

- Don't assume that a service user is wrong just because he or she has dementia.

- Don't patronise a service user with dementia or treat them like a child. Never refer to the person as a 'case', such as 'a stroke' or 'an Alzheimer's' or talk about them as if they weren't there.

Other sources of support

- Check out what help the service user already receives and discuss with their family and your supervisor whether there are any other sources of support they could access, such as church groups, local voluntary services etc.

Record keeping

- Make a record of the service user's needs, preferences and care and support you provide for them. Your supervisor will be monitoring the service user's progress and you can refer to the notes when you report to your supervisor, either during your regular meetings or if you have particular concerns.

Other possible causes of confusion and memory problems

There are other reasons why a person may become confused or lose their memory. Here are some examples.

- Physical illness. If a person suddenly becomes confused this may be due to an illness, such as a urinary tract infection or the flu. Sometimes called delirium, this sort of confusion is usually temporary.

- Dehydration is also a common cause of confusion.

- The side effects of certain drugs, such as sedatives or some treatments for Parkinson's disease.

- Mental illness. Some forms of mental illness, such as schizophrenia, can cause what seems to be confusion or strange behaviour. Depression or stress can contribute to a poor memory.

- Vitamin B1 deficiency, which may occur because of a digestive problem.

- A long-term alcohol problem.

- A tumour. Pressure on the brain from a tumour or growth may result in confusion or unusual behaviour.

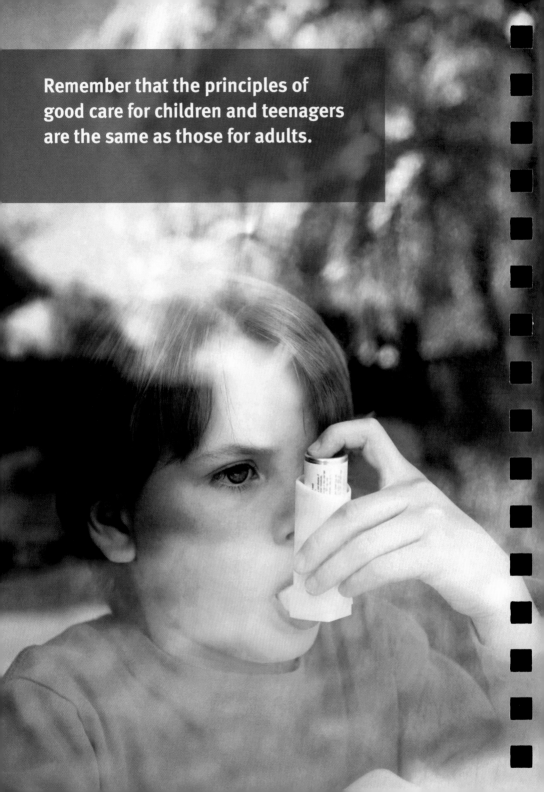

Remember that the principles of good care for children and teenagers are the same as those for adults.

12 Supporting children and young people

Care work with children and young people is based on the same principles as care work with adults. However, there are two important differences.

- Before visiting young service users, your employer will need to apply for an appropriate disclosure check to make sure there is nothing in your background that prevents you from working with children. This may be in addition to the checks required for working with vulnerable adults.

- Confidentiality policies and procedures may be different when working with children and young people. While their right to confidentiality should be respected, there may be certain types of information that you must pass on. For example if a young person tells you about something illegal or something that could cause harm to the young person or to others, you may need to report this. Seek guidance from your agency and read the relevant policies.

There are many reasons why a child or young person might need homecare support.

- The young person may have a long-term illness such as asthma or a terminal illness such as some types of cancer.

- There may be a need to support the family as a whole, or provide help and support for other children in the family.

- The parent or carer who usually looks after the child might be ill.

- The child may be home from boarding school because of holidays, an accident, sickness or school closure.

- You may be providing care for an adult who is usually looked after by a child or young person – so you will be working in partnership with the child or young person.

Supporting a child or young person

- Remember that the principles of good care for children and teenagers are the same as those for adults.

- Follow any instructions for specific care and support needs that are given by members of the paediatric homecare or child development teams.

- The care plan will have been agreed with the parent, ideally in consultation with the child. Therefore you'll need to take into account the wishes of the parent as well as the child.

- Seek specialist training and be aware of the policies and procedures relating to child abuse and protection.

Your relationship with the child or young person

- Find out about the development patterns that relate to the age group of the child or young person you are working with.

- Agree what you will call each other. For example does the child have a nickname, and would you prefer them to call you by your first name?

- If you are working with a younger child, think of games, rhymes, jokes etc that you can use to keep them amused.

- Talk to older children about their interests and listen to their ideas.

- Remember that you will be playing a part in the child's education and development.

- Be prepared to listen to the child or young person. Give straightforward responses, and remember that the principles of confidentiality apply to adolescents as well as adults.

- A child may feel comfortable telling you things that they wouldn't share with anyone else. Make sure the child knows that if they tell you about something that is illegal or about something that puts them or others at risk, you have a duty to pass that information on. Follow your agency's policies and procedures on this.

- Be consistent in your approach to children and young people.

- If the child or young person is unable to communicate using speech ask and find out about the ways in which they do communicate.

- Some of the words and terms used in care plans for children may be slightly different from those used for adults. Before you start working with a child read through the care plan and, if you're unsure of the meanings of any of the words or phrases, check these with your supervisor.

- If a child or adolescent provokes you, respond calmly and don't argue. It is usually unlawful to use any form of restraint or punishment.

Your relationship with parents and family members

- Be clear about your agency's relationship with the parents and make members of the family aware that you are working to your agency's policies and procedures.

- When you first start to work with a child, be prepared for the parents to check what you are doing and to see how the child reacts to you.

- You will probably have a better chance of forming a good relationship with a child if you can spend some time with them on their own (without the parent being there). Talk to the parent about how much time you will spend on your own with the child. This may depend on the child's age and the length of time you have worked with the family.

- Build appropriate relationships with other members of the family that you see often, such as the child's brothers and sisters.

- Be as open as possible with the child and the parent.

- While you are supporting a child, responsibility for that child is delegated to you. It is reasonable to expect the child to respond to your requests and behave in an acceptable way. If you have any problems, talk to the parent and other members of the child's support team.

- If you feel you are being asked to do things that are outside the care plan or go beyond the parent's agreement with the agency, talk to your supervisor about it.

- Support the child or young person's parents in their caring role.

- Don't get drawn into family relationships or issues that are outside the scope of your job.

- If you have concerns about the care the parents are giving to a child or young person you should refer to your agency's child protection policy.

Child protection

Agencies that work with children will have a specific policy relating to child protection. You will need to make sure that you have read and understood this and your role in ensuring the safety of children in your care. The policy will cover who you should report concerns to and other organisations that your employer might need to involve if issues or concerns arise.

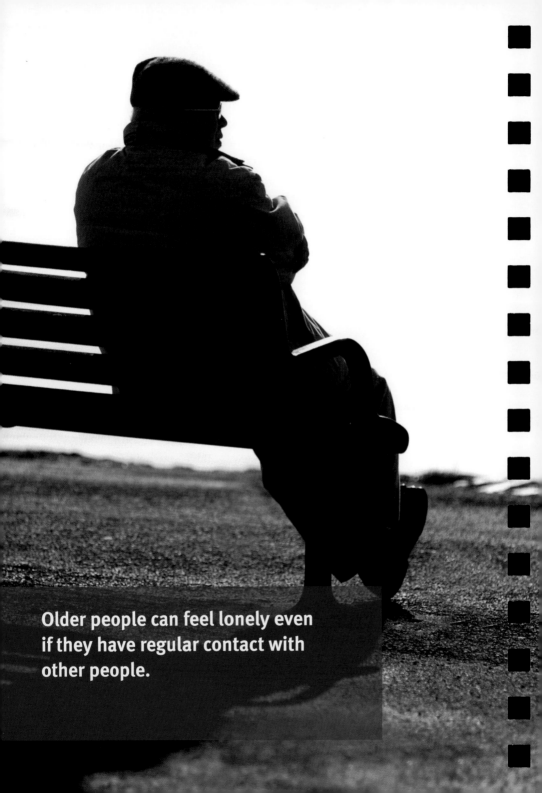

Older people can feel lonely even if they have regular contact with other people.

13 Supporting older people

The proportion of people over the age of 65 has grown steadily in the UK and is predicted to increase during the coming decades. The number of people living into their 80s and 90s is also increasing. While people's ideas about what 'old' means are changing, stereotypes about older people still exist. It is important to remember that older people are individuals with their own attitudes, abilities, interests and support needs.

Many of your service users will be older people, which is why much of the guidance in this handbook is directed towards caring for an older age group. This chapter focuses on the social aspects of your work and encourages you to think about your own ideas about older people.

The following issues can affect older people:

- Loneliness and isolation. Older people can feel lonely even if they have regular contact with other people. They may live alone, family members may live a long distance away or they may be missing loved ones who have died.

- Memory loss is not an inevitable part of ageing, but a person's chance of having memory problems increases with age. See *Chapter 11 – Supporting people with dementia* for more information.

- Depending on their personality, background and life experiences, some older people may hold opinions and beliefs that used to be common, but now seem out of date. They may find current attitudes, language or behaviour difficult to understand or find it unacceptable.

- There is a danger that older people may behave in a way that they think is expected of them – for example being 'grateful', not making a 'fuss' or not being too 'demanding'.

What you can do

- Take care not to stereotype older people. Treat each person as an individual.

- Treat all older people with dignity and respect and don't patronise them or treat them differently from other service users. Check their preferences and choices, and find out how they would like to be addressed and avoid terms like 'dear' or 'love', which are undignified.

- Encourage older service users who live alone to have contact with other people, if they would like to do this. Recognise that just because an older person has physical problems it doesn't mean their mental abilities are affected.

- Help older people to maintain their sense of independence by supporting them to carry out tasks rather than doing things for them.

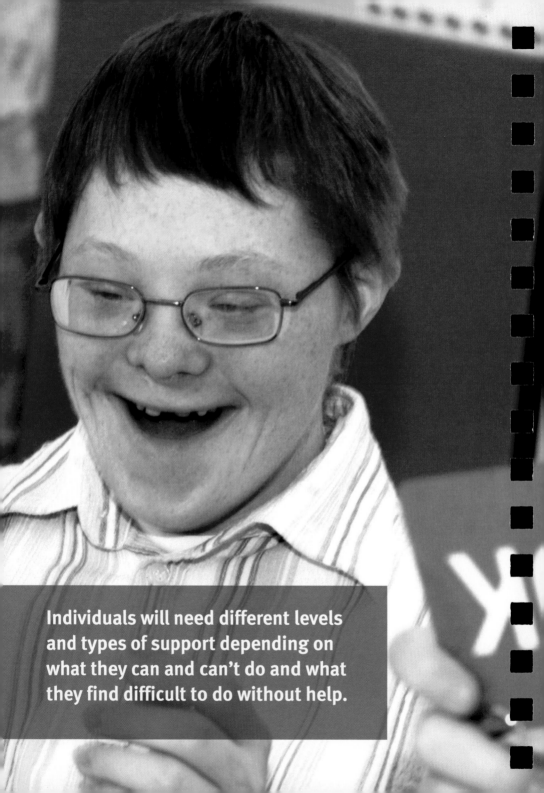

Individuals will need different levels and types of support depending on what they can and can't do and what they find difficult to do without help.

14 Supporting people with learning disabilities

With the right support, people with learning disabilities can live full and independent lives. When you are working with people with learning disabilities, remember the principles of good care. It is important to offer support that:

- Respects the rights of people with learning disabilities
- Treats them as individuals
- Enables them to live as independently as possible
- Empowers them to make choices
- Develops their skills
- Empowers them to be part of their community and have a social and family life

About learning disabilities

A person with a learning disability has reduced intellectual abilities and may have problems with everyday things such as socialising and doing household or financial tasks. Learning disabilities affect people throughout their lives. A person may have learning disabilities because:

- Something affected the development of their brain or spinal cord before they were born. For example their mother may have had an illness or accident during pregnancy.

- They were born prematurely.

- They didn't get enough oxygen during birth.

- Their brain was affected by an illness when they were a baby or young child.

- They have a genetic condition, such as Down's syndrome.

Learning disabilities covers a wide range of abilities from individuals who live and work independently but need support with some aspects of their life to those who have more complex disabilities and need support in many areas of their life. This means individuals will need different levels and types of support depending on their abilities and what they find difficult to do without help. Individuals with a learning disability may also have other difficulties such as vision, hearing, speech or mobility problems.

Remember that individuals with a learning disability using your services:

- Enjoy the same activities as other people.

- May take longer to learn, and may need additional support to develop new skills.

- May need support to complete certain tasks.

- May need support to help them make decisions. See *Chapter 9 – Mental health,* for more information about mental capacity and decision making.

- May experience difficulty with their emotions.

- May have problems with communication.

- May be too trusting of others, and unaware of dangers or inappropriate relationships.

- May be unaware of the boundaries of 'normal' social behaviour.

- May display behaviour that is challenging – for example they may become disruptive, if they are having difficulty being understood.

If you are supporting someone with a learning disability:

- Learn about the person as an individual - find out a little bit of history about the person, what they like and don't like, how they communicate etc. Speak to the individual's family, carers, friends, advocates (often referred to as significant others). Tailor the support you offer according to the individual's needs and preferences.

- Work closely with the individual's family carers, friends, advocates etc so that you are consistent in your approach to supporting them. Follow any established routines for basic skills such as washing, dressing, cooking and shopping.

- Support the development of the person's social skills.

- Encourage the individual to join in with any activities.

- Be prepared to help them to communicate and express his or her needs and feelings. This may involve learning techniques to help you communicate with them – for example if the person uses 'Makaton' you could learn the basics of Makaton. The techniques you develop will depend on the abilities of the individual.

- Provide relief and support for the primary carer – it may help them to share and discuss any issues or problems with you.

- Seek specialist training, supervision and support.

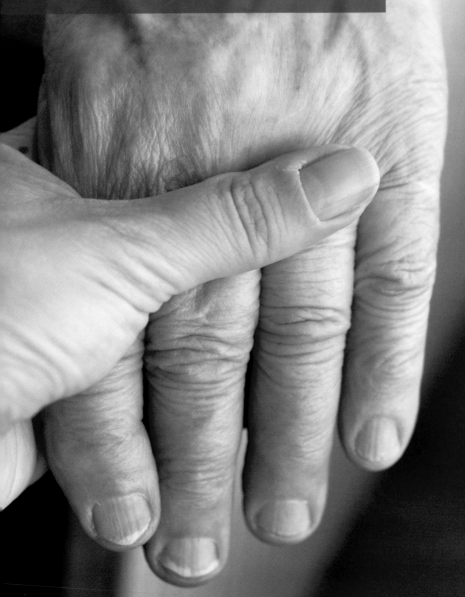

Physical touch can be very important, especially if people don't have family or friends around them. Just holding hands can be very comforting.

15   End of life care

You may work with a service user who is dying or within the final 12 months of life. This type of care is known as 'end of life care'. If you are involved in providing end of life care you are likely to be part of a team that may include specialist health and care professionals as well as the person's GP and their relatives.

Caring for someone who is dying may be emotionally challenging. However, it can also be rewarding to know that you have been able to offer the person and their family comfort and support during a distressing time.

As with all service users, you should:

- Treat them with dignity and respect.

- Support people to make decisions about their care at the end of life wherever possible.

- Provide care in a way that takes into account their wishes, culture and background.

- Be prepared to provide support that can change rapidly according to the person's condition.

What happens when a person is dying?

The symptoms that occur at the end of life will vary from person to person. The person may:

- Sleep more and more, or be unable to sleep

- Be in pain

- Lose the desire to eat or drink

- Feel sick or be sick

- Find it difficult to swallow, or have a very dry mouth

- Lose control of their bowel or bladder, or have constipation

- Find it harder to breathe because of a build up of fluid in the lung – their breathing may be noisy

- Feel cold, or their skin may become cold to the touch

- Become confused or agitated.

Your role

- To continue to provide safe, dignified and effective care that responds to the service user's needs.

- Observe changes in the health of service users and be able to recognise any signs and symptoms that could indicate that they are approaching the end of their life.

- Know who the members of the person's end-of-life care team are and who you should contact if there is a change in the person's condition.

- Know who has Power of Attorney (if there is someone) in case the person loses the capacity to make decisions for themselves.

Understanding the person and their wishes

- Find out as much as you can about the service user's state of health and the support they need. You can find this out from the service user themselves, or from your supervisor and the person's family.

- Make sure you are aware of the person's end of life care plan. This may include information about psychological, spiritual and cultural needs as well as their health and care needs.

- Be aware of any wishes and preferences the service user has previously expressed (your supervisor will tell you if there is a valid "advance care plan" or "advance statement" in place). If they discuss any new needs or wishes, bring them to the attention of the appropriate person if you have the service user's permission to do so.

- Be ready for the possibility that a person may want to talk about their death and the plans for their care. Think about your role in these discussions – is it appropriate for you to help the person to make plans for their future care, or does the person just want someone to listen? It may be appropriate to refer the person to another professional or a family member.

- Do not put pressure on a service user to have these discussions, but offer support and advice if you are asked.

- Encourage service users to contribute to plans about their care for as long as they are able to do so.

- If the service user wishes it, be open in your discussions with their friends and relatives about the approaching death.

Physical support

- Try to make sure that the person is physically comfortable.

- Support the person as you would any other service user. Don't be tempted to 'take over'.

- Note anything you observe about the service user, such as the skin (colour, tone and dryness), breathing and drug routines.

- Be aware of any specific drug regime or equipment that is introduced as a person's condition changes. Make sure you are trained to use any new equipment.

- Follow instructions given by other members of the care team. Recording fluid intake is very important towards end of life, to maintain hydration and avoid confusion.

- If the person no longer wants to drink, they may find it refreshing if you wipe around their mouth with a swab dipped in clean water. Swabbing the person's mouth with glycerine can also help to relieve a dry mouth.

- Medication is a significant part of end of life care, to control pain and other unpleasant symptoms. Late or missed doses of medication can be extremely distressing and increases a person's pain unnecessarily.

- Meals can be an important part of everyone's day. People at the end of life can experience appetite loss, nausea or difficulty eating. Try and find foods that the person can eat and enjoy, even if they only manage small quantities. Meal replacement drinks may also form part of the person's diet.

Recognising pain

- If the person can no longer communicate easily, observe them carefully and look out for signs of pain. For example, someone who is in pain might:

  - make noises, such as whimpering or groaning

  - have a distorted facial expression

  - have changing breathing patterns – for example short periods when they breathe rapidly or noisily

  - become pale or have clammy skin

- If you think a service user is in pain, report it to the appropriate person – if you are not sure who this is, ask your supervisor.

Emotional support

- Be straightforward with the service user – for example don't talk about getting better if the person has accepted that this is not possible. Be as 'normal' as you can in your conversation and in the way you treat the person.

- If the person wants to talk about their pain, or fears and anxieties about dying, encourage this and don't deny that they exist.

- Be prepared to listen to stories about the past and special memories, even if you have heard them before. Telling these stories may give real pleasure to the service user.

- If it does not cause pain, physical touch can be very important to someone who is dying, especially if they don't have family or friends around them. Just holding hands can be very comforting.

- Respect the person's need to withdraw from social contact.

Find out from the service user or their family about any spiritual, religious or cultural considerations the person would want to be taken into account.

Supporting the person's family

- Respect the knowledge of family members and treat them as partners in the person's care.

- Be prepared to help family members to understand the physical changes that take place at the end of life.

- Be ready to listen if family members want to talk about their feelings. Listen without passing judgement or offering advice, unless you are asked to.

- Relatives may feel helpless or useless – you could suggest things for them to do that would help them and the service user.

- Your supervisor will tell you how the process of verification and certification of death works in your area, so that you can advise the family if needed.

Looking after yourself

- Seek specialist training on end of life care and make sure you receive regular supervision.

- Acknowledge your own feelings about looking after someone who is dying. Talk about your feelings to colleagues, your supervisor or in training.

- If you feel upset after someone has died, make sure you discuss this with your supervisor. You may need bereavement support yourself.

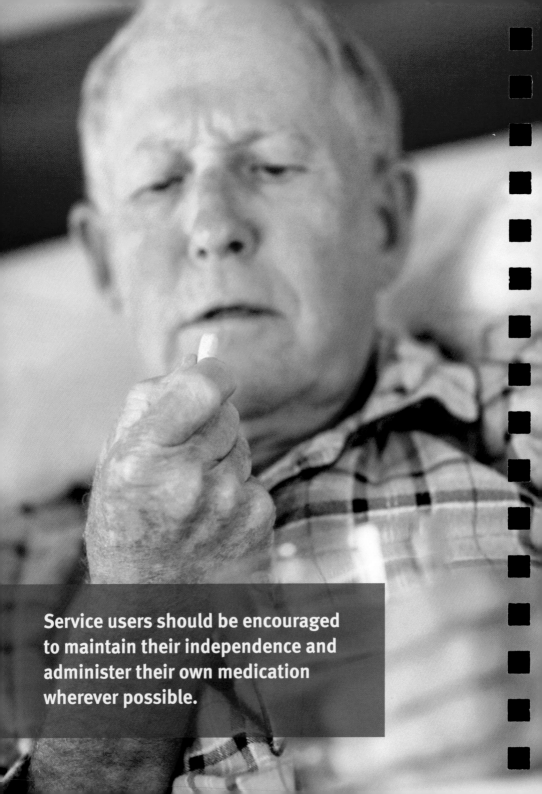

Service users should be encouraged to maintain their independence and administer their own medication wherever possible.

16   Helping service users with medication

Your role may include supporting service users to take medication. This chapter gives some general guidelines, however it is essential to follow your agency's policy and procedures on medication/medicines.

When helping service users with medication, remember the principles of good practice. You must maintain service users' right to privacy, dignity and choice. Service users should be encouraged to maintain their independence and administer their own medication wherever possible. Recording of medication is extremely important, to avoid medicines being given more than once (particularly if several careworkers or family members are involved in assisting with medicines) and to check back if there is a problem.

Types of medication

If you have had the appropriate level of training, you may be asked to support a service user with the following types of medication:

- Prescription medication – medicines that are prescribed by a qualified health professional, such as a GP, hospital doctor, specialist nurse or dentist.

- Controlled drugs – these are prescribed medicines that are subject to additional controls under the Misuse of Drugs Act. Your agency should have special rules and guidance relating to controlled drugs.

- Over the counter (OTC) medication – medicines, lotions etc that can be bought from a pharmacist, supermarket or other retail outlet.

- 'As and when required' (PRN – from the latin 'pro re nata') medication – this is medicine that a service user may need to take occasionally when they need it, rather than in regular doses (see below).

To support a service user with any of the following, you must have received specialist training:

- Eye, ear and nose drops.

- Inhalers, nebulisers and oxygen.

- Injections, enemas or suppositories.

- Emergency PRN medication.

- Any form of medication that involves skilled observations to be made before, during or after administration.

If you have any doubts about your ability to assist a service user with their medication, or are worried that you haven't had the right training, seek advice from your supervisor.

Your employer's policies and procedures

Your agency or employer should have policies and procedures that cover the following issues related to medication – make sure you are aware of their content and what you may and may not do according to these policies:

- Safe administration of medication

- Purchasing OTC medication and assisting service users with this kind of medication.

- Obtaining prescriptions on behalf of a service user.

- Identifying how service users give consent to take medication.

- Supporting a service user with PRN medication.

- Storage and safekeeping of medicines.

- Management of controlled medicines.

- Disposal of unwanted/expired medicines.

- Record keeping.

- Incident reporting (eg overdoses, missed doses and wrong doses).

Assessment and recording

An assessment will have been made of the service user's medication needs, including the type of support a careworker should give and how the service user will give their consent to medication. This information should be included in the service user's care plan.

A medication administration record (MAR) should also be drawn up and kept in the service user's home as part of the care plan. You will use the MAR to note the details each time you support a service user with their medication.

What you may be required to do

Depending on the level of training you have received, you may be asked to do one or more of the following:

- If the person is independent they may only need physical assistance with their medication. If they request it, care staff might help a service user to take their medication, for example opening bottles and packets; shaking bottles; removing lids from bottles; popping pills out of packages; pouring out medicine.

- If the person can manage their medication but needs reminders or prompts, then care staff might need to give a verbal reminder to take medication at the correct time or ask if they have taken their medication.

- If the person cannot manage their medication needs on their own you may be required to check the medication that is required against the service user's medication administration (MAR) record, pouring a measured dose into a container for them to swallow, physically giving the medication, applying cream or ointment to the skin, administering eye, ear or nose drops, or giving invasive medications such as injections or suppositories. How much assistance you give will depend on what you have been trained to do and on your agency's policies and procedures.

If you are required to support a service user with their medication, remember the following:

- Be aware of policies and procedures to ensure the safe administration of medication.

- It is A LEGAL REQUIREMENT that you follow the prescriber's instructions, which are usually written on the medication label. If the service user uses a monitored dosage system provided by a pharmacist (this is an aid with compartments that contain pills to be taken at different times each day) it should come with details of all medication contained in the system. If you are unsure about any aspect of the instructions, discuss this with your supervisor or the prescriber.

- Keep information about a service user's treatment and medication confidential.

- Attend training as required by your employer. Ask for training if you don't feel confident with any aspect of your role.

- Keep accurate records.

Checking the medication

The 5 "rights" of medication administration

1. The **right dose** of

2. The **right medicine**

3. Given to the **right person**

4. At the **right time**

5. By the **right route**.

- Check the correct dose by looking at the medication label and the medication administration record. Measure out the correct dose, using a measuring container or measuring spoon if appropriate. If you think a pre-measured dosage system would help the service user to take the correct dose, discuss this with your supervisor or the pharmacist.

- Check on the MAR that it is the right time for the service user to take the medication.

- Check the original container for the name of the service user. Medication must only be administered to the person it was prescribed for.

- If using a monitored dosage system, only administer medication from the correct compartment. Only use a dosage system that has been prepared by a pharmacist.

- Check that the medication is within the expiry date given on the packaging.

- Check against the MAR that it is the right type of medication.

- Make sure you are giving the medication by the right route.

- Check that the service user hasn't already taken the medication, by asking the service user and looking at the MAR.

Supporting the service user to take the medication

- Some religious practices, such as fasting, may affect the timing of a service user's medication. In this situation, follow guidance given by the prescriber.

- The service user should be sitting or standing in order to swallow medicine or pills. Unless you are trained to do so, do not give medication to someone who is lying down.

- Prepare a drink for the service user – ideally a glass of water – if they need it to take the medication. Follow any instructions about what the medication should be taken with. For example, some medicines should not be taken with certain drinks such as milk or grapefruit juice.

- Encourage the service user to follow instructions about what to eat and drink while taking prescribed medicines.

- If the service user refuses to take medication or is unable to take it, make a note of this in the MAR and follow your agency's policy and procedures.

- Tell your supervisor about any changes in the service user's ability to take their medication.

Some things you should NEVER do

- If you miss a dose, don't give a double dose next time. Record the missed dose in the service user's records and report it to your supervisor straight away, so they can seek advice from the PRESCRIBER if necessary.

- Don't put out medication for a service user or someone else to administer later.

- Never crush tablets or open capsules. This is likely to affect the way the medication works. Check this with the prescriber or pharmacist if necessary. They may be able to provide a soluble or liquid form of the medication instead.

- Never force anyone to take medication against their will.

- Don't administer medicines from an unsealed compliance aid filled by a service user's relatives. It is safer to do so from the original containers, because they will have information about the timing, dosage instructions etc.

- If any medication is dropped on the floor, don't give it to the service user. Make a note in the records, and follow any relevant disposal procedures. Dropped, refused or spat-out medication should be returned to the pharmacist for disposal.

- Never offer, sell, give advice on or recommend any form of medication, remedy or preparation, including homeopathic and herbal remedies.

'As and when required' (PRN) medication

Service users take this sort of medication when they feel they need it. (PRN stands for 'pro re nata', which means 'when required'.) You might play a role in helping the service user to take the medication, but they will make the decision about when it is necessary. Information about the frequency and maximum dosage should be on the medication container and the MAR.

Always record that a service user has taken a PRN medicine, including the dose and time it was taken, so that careworkers visiting later know what the service user has taken.

Some PRN medicines are for use in an emergency, when the service user might be unable to request them. You should be given special training if you are likely to be required to administer PRN medicines under these circumstances, and the particular situations where this might be necessary will be clearly described in the care plan.

Over the counter (OTC) medication

Service users may wish to use over the counter (OTC) medication, for example painkillers or skin creams, for minor ailments.

If your role includes buying OTC medication on behalf of a service user, you should not make the decision about what type of medication to buy. This decision should be made by the service user, prescriber or pharmacist, depending on the circumstances.

If a service user is considering taking an OTC drug they haven't used before, ensure this is agreed by the PRESCRIBER in case it interacts with medication they are already taking.

If your role involves helping a service user to take OTC medication, make a note of the dose, timing and type of medication in the medication administration record (MAR), as you would with prescription medicines.

Assisting children with medication

Usually parents will administer medication to children, but a careworker might be asked to do this under some circumstances. If you are required to do this, you should be given specific training to learn about dosage sizes and methods of administration for children. Children generally need much smaller doses of medication than adults.

Hiding medication (covert administration)

Usually service users are only assisted with medication with their consent. However, occasionally a service user who is unable to make an informed decision about whether to take medication (for example someone with dementia) may refuse to take it. In this situation, the person's 'best interests' will be decided by people close to the service user, such as family members, doctors, nursing staff, or someone who has been given legal powers to make decisions on behalf of the service user. If it is agreed that it is in the service user's best interests to take the medication, you will receive guidance on what medication to give and how to give it. This may mean giving the medication covertly, ie without the service user's knowledge. There are many potential problems with covert administration and it should not be undertaken without careful planning.

Record keeping

The administration of all medication, lotions and creams should be recorded on a service user's medication administration record. This includes details of all medication given from a monitored dosage system. If a service user refuses to take medication, or if they have any side effects, or it has been given by someone else, such as a family member or day centre, this should also be recorded.

Always treat records of a service user's medication as confidential.

Reporting errors and incidents

If something goes wrong with a service user's medication, it is vital for their health and wellbeing that you report and record this in line with your agency's procedures. It is always better to report a medication error than to try and hide it.

An error or incident could include:

- Missed doses.
- Giving medicine at the wrong time.
- Administration of too much or too little medication.
- Administration of the wrong type of medication.
- Medication taken the wrong way, for example if the service user swallows a skin cream.
- Medication given to the wrong person.

If this happens:

- Follow your agency's accident and incident reporting procedure.

- If the person becomes ill, apply emergency first aid if needed or call the emergency services. Do not try to make the service user be sick.

- Contact your supervisor straight away, so that they can review what has happened and notify external organisations (eg a GP where appropriate).

- Record the error or incident in the service user's records. This should include what was given/taken or omitted, when this took place, the dosage given, any changes in the service user's condition and any emergency action taken.

Storage and disposal of medicine

- Make sure medicines, pills and creams/lotions are stored in the correct conditions. Most need to be stored in a cool, dry place, but check the label in case other conditions apply.

- Keep medicines in a safe place that is known to the service user and other carers.

- The safest way to dispose of medicine is to return it in its container to the pharmacy. This is usually the service user's responsibility, unless another arrangement has been agreed with the agency.

- If you are required to dispose of medicine, record this according to your agency's procedures. This may include getting the service user's signature to show that they consented to the disposal. For controlled drugs, you may also need to get a signature from the pharmacist who takes the unwanted medication for disposal.

- Don't put unwanted medicines in with the household rubbish or put them down the sink or toilet.

- If a service user dies, follow your agency's procedures regarding disposal of unused medicines. If the death is referred to the coroner, medication will need to be kept in case the coroner needs to see it. Once the death certificate has been issued, it can then be disposed of in the normal way.

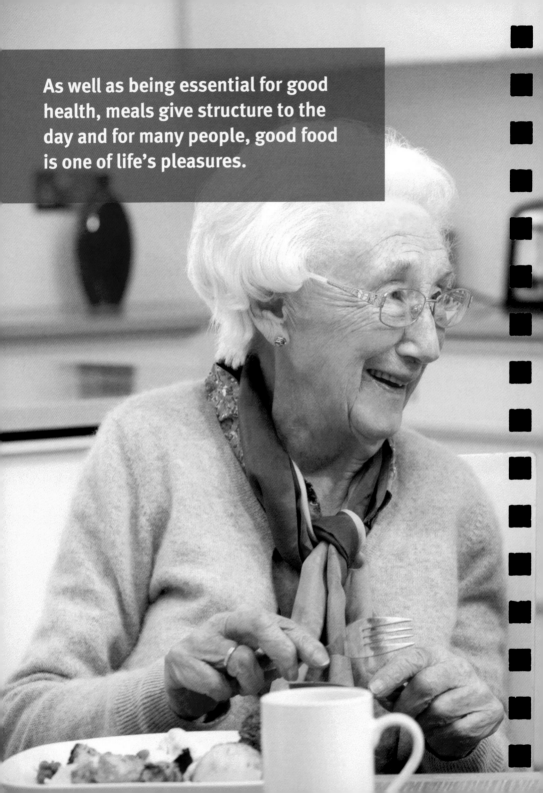

As well as being essential for good health, meals give structure to the day and for many people, good food is one of life's pleasures.

17 Food and nutrition

Food is an important part of our lives. A balanced diet that gives us all of the nutrients we need is vital to maintain health and wellbeing. As well as being essential for good health, meals give structure to the day and for many people, good food is one of life's pleasures.

Eating the vitamins and minerals found in a healthy and balanced diet helps us fight off illnesses and recover more quickly when we do get ill. Eating enough protein helps build and maintain muscles and sufficient carbohydrates provide energy for activity.

If you are involved in planning and preparing meals for service users, it is important to make sure that they get the essential nutrients and fluids they need. You should make sure that you respect their choices and understand their dietary needs and physical ability to eat, as well as their cultural preferences. Try to make meal times as pleasant as possible.

Even if planning and preparing meals isn't one of your duties, you will need to be able to understand where a person might be at risk of malnutrition and recognise possible signs that they may need additional support.

Malnutrition

Malnutrition occurs when a person doesn't get enough nutrients, or doesn't get the right balance of nutrients needed for good health. Although weight loss can be a sign that someone is malnourished, it is not the case that only thin or underweight people are malnourished. It is possible to have a diet that is high in calories but low in some or most of the vitamins and minerals that the body needs, this means that someone who is overweight could also be suffering from malnutrition.

People can be at risk of malnutrition for a number of reasons. They may find cooking difficult because of a physical disability, eating might be difficult because of painful teeth, a painful mouth or their ability to swallow may be limited. People who live alone and are socially isolated or who have mobility/transport issues are also at risk. Some medical conditions can also make a person more prone to malnutrition such as dementia (forgetting to eat or unable to communicate their needs), persistent vomiting or diarrhoea, or cancer and other diseases which can cause a loss of appetite.

Symptoms of malnutrition can include:

- Weight loss
- Tiredness/fatigue
- Muscle wasting
- Dry skin
- Irritability
- Delayed recovery from illness
- Increased susceptibility to illness
- Brittle nails
- Dizziness
- Diarrhoea
- Skin rashes
- Swollen tongue/sore mouth

Dehydration

Dehydration occurs when the body loses more fluids than it is taking in and stops the body from functioning normally. This can happen because a person is not drinking enough fluids or because they are losing more fluid from the body than usual, perhaps due to sweating during exercise or in hot weather, vomiting or diarrhoea. Some medical conditions such as diabetes or alcoholism can also cause dehydration.

To prevent dehydration it is recommended that a person drinks about 1.2 litres of fluid every day. This works out to be about six 200ml or eight 150ml glasses. You can help your service users remain properly hydrated by making sure they have access to hot and cold drinks through the day, making sure they are given a drink at meal times and looking for signs that they may be becoming dehydrated. Some foods, such as fruit and vegetables, are also high in water content and can be beneficial in ensuring adequate fluid intake.

Symptoms of dehydration

- Thirst
- Dark coloured and strong smelling urine
- Dizziness
- Tiredness
- Dry mouth or lips
- Infrequent urination
- Dry skin

If untreated, dehydration can become severe and may cause symptoms such as:

- Confusion
- Low blood pressure
- Weak pulse
- Rapid heartbeat
- Low level of consciousness
- Fits

Long-term dehydration can affect kidney function and cause kidney stones to develop. It can also cause constipation, liver and muscle damage and problems with cholesterol.

If someone is dehydrated their fluid levels will need replenishing. Where someone is finding it difficult to keep liquids down try giving a small amount but frequently through the day.

If you suspect that someone is severely dehydrated you should report it to your agency so that medical advice can be sought.

Healthy eating

A varied and balanced diet containing the right proportions of the five food groups listed below will ensure that the service user gets all the nutrients they need.

A diet based on starchy foods such as rice and pasta; with plenty of fruit and vegetables; some protein-rich foods such as meat, fish and lentils; some milk and dairy foods; and not too much fat, salt or sugar, will give you all the nutrients you need. In general around one-third of a meal should be from group 1, one-third from group 2 and the rest mainly from groups 3 and 4 with group 5 being kept to only a small proportion of the meal.

The five food groups

1. Fruit and vegetables

These are a vital part of any diet and we should eat 5 portions a day. Eating different coloured fruit and vegetables will provide a wider variety of nutrients.

2. Bread, rice, pasta, potatoes and other starchy food

These are a good source of energy. Wholemeal or wholegrain varieties contain more fibre and usually more vitamins and minerals than white varieties.

3. Meat, eggs, fish and pulses.

These are all good sources of protein and help the body to repair cells and tissues.

4. Milk and dairy

These are also good sources of protein but choose lower fat options such as semi-skimmed or skimmed milk if fat content is an issue.

5. Food and drink high in fat and/or sugar

While too much fat can be bad for you, some fat is needed for energy and to help with vitamin absorption.

Definitions

Fat

There are two types of fat:

- Saturated fat – found in foods such as pies, butter, full-cream, cakes, cheese and biscuits. Eating too much saturated fat can raise cholesterol levels and can lead to conditions such as high blood pressure, heart disease and stroke.

- Unsaturated fat – found in fish, avocados, vegetable oils, nuts and seeds. A small amount of unsaturated fat a day can help lower cholesterol and help to keep us healthy.

Carbohydrates

Carbohydrates provide the body with energy. There are two types:

- Complex carbohydrates found in starchy foods such as those listed in Group 1 which are good for you.

- Simple carbohydrates found in cakes, biscuits, cereals and puddings which would fall into Group 5. These are not so good for you and should be eaten in small amounts.

Fibre

Fibre keeps the digestive system healthy – there are two types:

- Insoluble fibre found in grains, wholemeal bread, cereals, pasta, vegetable and fruit that contains seeds – helps prevent constipation and bowel problems.

- Soluble fibre found in all fruits and vegetables – lowers cholesterol and controls blood sugar.

Protein

Protein is needed for growth and cell repair and is also a good source of energy. It can be found in meat, fish, eggs, beans, cereals, nuts and pulses.

Vitamins and minerals

There are two main types of vitamins. "Fat-soluble" vitamins are stored in the body while "water-soluble" vitamins are not.

A balanced diet containing fresh fruit and vegetables, meat, fish, dairy products and grains (bread, pasta and rice) will provide all the necessary vitamins and minerals.

Planning healthy meals

If you are involved in menu planning, shopping or preparing meals for a service user, it is important to:

- Treat the service user with sensitivity and respect – for example by respecting their choices and preferences, ensuring a pleasant environment in which to eat, giving them enough time for meals and giving assistance in a sensitive way.

- Consider the mental capacity of the service user. Information in the care plan about the person's likes and dislikes will help you to make an appropriate decision on their behalf if they are not able to choose for themselves.

- Take the service user's nutritional state into account – for example whether they are overweight or underweight.

- Bear in mind any cultural preferences and religious requirements – for example halal or kosher food are important religious observances, while other people may make a choice to be vegetarian or avoid certain foods.

- Consider any medical and special dietary needs. These will have been identified in the service user's assessment. Strictly follow any special diets or other guidance.

- Make sure meals have the right balance of nutrients and food groups.

- Think about the timing of meals. What time does the service user prefer to eat and drink? If there are long periods between visits, it may be necessary to leave food and drink for the person to eat during the day.

Menu planning

- Wherever possible, plan menus with the service user or their family members.

- Include plenty of variety – avoid repeating meals from day-to-day but if the person has a particular 'routine', help them to maintain it.

- Avoid using similar ingredients or cooking styles from day-to-day – for example don't serve two beef dishes or two microwaved dishes on consecutive days.

- Do not assume that people always follow the dietary requirements of their cultural background or religion and meet the needs of those who do. If in doubt ask about the person's preferences sensitively.

- Make sure the meals you plan are not beyond the cooking skills of other careworkers.

- Make sure meals can be prepared within the allocated time.

- Include different textures within each meal.

- Plan meals that will look attractive, with different coloured foods on the plate.

- Change menus to reflect the seasons, for example lighter meals or salads in summer and warming food in winter.

- Don't forget drinks.

- Make sure portion size is consistent – where possible, discuss with the service user the quantity of food they prefer.

- The temperature that food is served at is important for food hygiene and the enjoyment of meals. Be careful to get the temperature right.

Special dietary needs

Service users with certain health conditions or allergies may have to avoid certain foods or eat at regular times. Always check each service user's care plan for their individual dietary needs.

Food shopping

- Use the menu plan to make a shopping list. Involve the service user in this process if possible.

- Check 'use by' and 'best before' dates of foods, bearing in mind the week's menu plan. 'Use by' dates are put on food that can go off quickly. These foods should be eaten on or before the date shown. 'Best before' dates are put onto food that has a longer shelf life. The date indicates when it is at its best quality. Once the date has been passed, the food will start to deteriorate and so should be eaten as soon as possible after this date.

- When shopping, buy frozen and chilled food last so it doesn't defrost or become warm.

- Keep raw and cooked foods separate.

- Pack food that could easily be crushed or damaged on top of other items.

- Don't put food near the heater in the car when taking it back to the service user's home.

Food storage

Fridge/freezer

- Put frozen or refrigerated food away within two hours of purchase or even sooner if the weather is hot.

- Check 'use by' and 'best before' dates of food and make sure anything that is past it's 'use by' date is thrown away. 'Best before' dates are put onto food that has a longer shelf life. The date indicates when it is at its best quality. Food can be eaten after this date but the product will start to deteriorate so the quality will not be as good as when initially purchased. Arrange food in the fridge so that foods which need to be eaten soonest are at the front.

- Store uncooked meats on a plate and put them on a lower shelf than cooked meat, so that fluids from one food cannot drip onto another.

- Store cheese in an airtight container, or wrap it well.

- Store salads and vegetables in a salad box.

- Cover liquids with a lid or cling film to prevent them absorbing odours or flavours from other foods.

- Cover unpackaged food so that it doesn't dry out.

- Always throw away food that looks rotten, smells and/or tastes bad, or has leaked out of its original container prior to opening.

- Regularly wipe the inside of the fridge.

Cupboards

- Where possible, put heavier jars and tins on the lowest shelves.

- Check cupboards for dampness, especially those used for dry foods.

- Keep ventilation openings clear.

- Store similar foods together.

- Throw away tins that are rusty, bulging or misshapen.

- Arrange food in cupboards, so that items which need to be used first are at the front.

Preparing and cooking food safely

If your role includes preparing meals for service users, you should have received food hygiene training. If you are unsure about any aspect of food hygiene or how to prepare meals safely, talk to your supervisor.

Preparation

- Remove any pets from the kitchen, remove cleaning products and materials from the food preparation area and put on some protective clothing.

- Before (and after) preparing food, wash your hands.

- Keep food preparation areas and equipment such as chopping boards, knives and bowls clean.

- Wash fruit and vegetables in clean water to remove any soil, chemicals and insects.

- Defrost frozen foods thoroughly before cooking them, unless they are supposed to be cooked from frozen. Plan ahead so that food is taken out of the freezer in good time to defrost.

- Keep raw food and cooked foods separate. In particular, keep raw meat, poultry and fish away from cooked meats.

- Don't use the same knife or chopping board to chop raw food, particularly meat, and cooked food. Wash utensils in hot soapy water and dry them with a clean cloth after using them for raw food and before using them for cooked food.

- Never put cooked food onto a plate that has been used for raw meat, poultry or fish without washing it first.

Cooking

- Cooking food at a temperature of at least 70°C and maintaining this temperature for at least two minutes will ensure that any harmful bacteria in the food are killed.

- Always follow the cooking instructions and cooking temperatures if they are given on the packet.

- Always pre-heat the oven or grill so that they are at the correct cooking temperature when you put the food in.

- Ensure meat such as pork and poultry is not pink or red at its thickest part, as this means it is not fully cooked. To check that meat is cooked, put a skewer into the centre (or thickest part) of the meat – if the juices run clear this usually means it is cooked. Alternatively, use a meat thermometer to tell you if the food has reached the required temperature.

- If serving meat rare, make sure the outside of the meat is fully cooked by sealing or searing it first (cooking the outside surfaces in a pan with some oil).

- When cooking fish, test the fish next to the bone – if it is opaque (ie no longer slightly transparent-looking) it is cooked. Some fish, such as salmon or tuna, can be eaten rare as long as they are sealed or seared first (see above).

- Raw shellfish will change colour during cooking. For example, uncooked prawns will go from grey to pink when cooked, and scallops will turn a milky white colour when cooked.

- Ensure liquid dishes such as soup simmer for at least two minutes.

- Eggs can contain harmful bacteria, such as salmonella, if they are not cooked thoroughly. It is best to avoid giving service users meals in which eggs are only lightly cooked, such as soft-boiled eggs.

- Pulses, such as kidney or butter beans, contain harmful toxins that are destroyed by the cooking process. It is safer to use tinned varieties, which are cooked before canning.

- Don't leave cooked or raw food at room temperature for longer than 90 minutes.

- Never store or refrigerate partially cooked food. Allow cooked food to cool to room temperature before putting it in the fridge.

- If you need to reheat food, make sure it is piping hot all the way through. Do not reheat cooked food more than once.

- When using a microwave, cover food so that it stays moist and to stop it splashing when you take it out. Follow the manufacturer's instructions where possible regarding the timing, microwave power and, for example, whether to make holes in the film lid.

- DO NOT use metal dishes in a microwave.

Food Hygiene

Raw food can be contaminated with bacteria so care must be taken to ensure it is purchased, stored, prepared and cooked correctly.

Any careworker who handles food must attend a food hygiene course relevant to the care they are providing. This will give information about how to handle food safely.

There should be a separate food hygiene policy within your organisation to refer to.

In brief, food handling can be made safer by making sure you follow the guidance below:

- Wash your hands before and after handling food, in between handling raw and cooked food, and after using the toilet, blowing the nose, touching the face and hair, touching pets or disposing of rubbish.

- Wash all fruit and vegetables.

- Use separate utensils and implements when handling raw and cooked foods (or thoroughly clean these between use).

- Store raw and cooked foods separately in the fridge.

- Keep food covered when being refrigerated.

- Clean work surfaces and any equipment used thoroughly after preparing food.

Meal times

The service user's care plan will include arrangements for mealtimes which have been agreed with the service user and/or their family members. Wherever possible, support service users to follow their usual routines, for example, sitting at the table to eat or having what they like to drink during or after a meal.

Make sure you follow any instructions on:

- When the service user likes to eat.

- Where the service user likes to eat.

- Other preferences such as whether the service user likes to have a napkin, what they like to drink with meals etc.

- Their position during the meal.

- Whether they like to have company while they eat.

Presentation

Good presentation makes food more attractive and enjoyable, and will encourage service users to eat. This is particularly important if they have a small appetite or are undernourished or dehydrated.

- Serve meals that service users are familiar with and like.

- Strong-smelling food, such as strong fish, can be off-putting – warn service users if you are going to cook something with a strong smell.

- Make sure food is well-cooked and looks tempting on the plate. Avoid combining foods that don't normally go together.

- Make sure salt, pepper and other seasonings or sauces are available.

- Plan meals that are colourful – a plateful of foods that are all the same colour will look boring.

- Serve food as soon as it has been cooked – as well as being more appetising, it will prevent bacteria from developing.

- Use garnishes such as a sprinkling of herbs or a lemon slice to make food more attractive.

- Make sure portions are the right size – too much or too little food on the plate can be off-putting.

- Use a plate that is a suitable size so that the meal isn't falling off the edge.

- Make sure plates, cups, cutlery etc are clean, and use the person's preferred crockery and cutlery.

- Before serving the meal, wipe away any drips on the plate that might make the meal look messy or sloppy.

- Don't forget to serve a drink with food.

- Remember that presentation is just as important for service users who are on a soft or liquid diet. Soft foods such as mashed potato can still be recognisable, and should be presented attractively in the ways listed above. If the service user drinks liquid foods, serve it in attractive glasses and at their preferred temperature.

- Allow service users the time they need to eat their meal. If they feel hurried they may be reluctant to eat.

Before eating

- People may like to wash their hands before meals.

- Some people will need to put their dentures in if they don't wear them all the time.

After eating

- When a service user has finished eating, clear away the crockery and cutlery and wipe up any spilled food.

- If a service user has spilled food down themselves, offer to help them to clean it up.

- They may wish to wash their hands, brush their teeth or clean their dentures.

Record keeping

It is important to keep food records for each service user. This should include records of menus, shopping, daily choices, what they have eaten and drunk and any assistance you have given. This will help to build up a picture of the service user's nutritional intake over time.

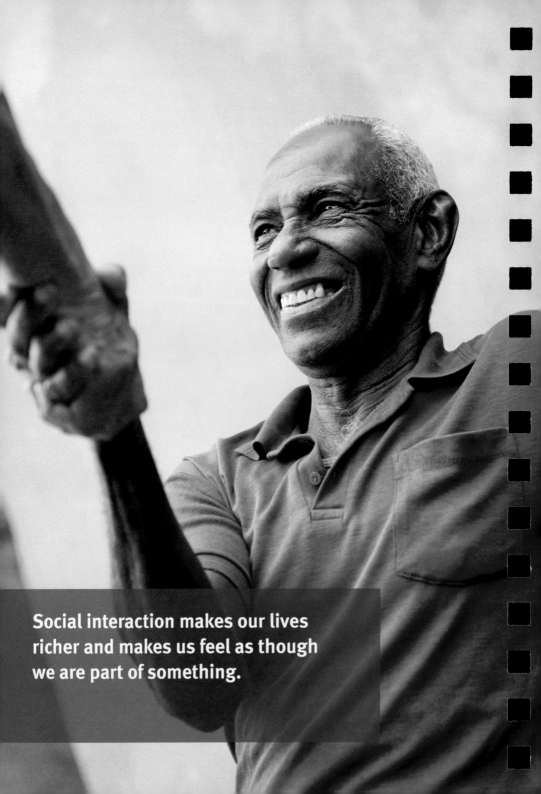

Social interaction makes our lives richer and makes us feel as though we are part of something.

18 Social and cultural life

Most of us enjoy contact with other people. From having lunch with old friends to a chat with the local shopkeeper, social interaction makes our lives richer and makes us feel as though we are part of something. It gives us the chance to laugh, explore our interests or share our problems, and it makes the routine things in life more enjoyable. An active social life is good for people's physical and mental health.

A service user's health, physical disability, or state of mind may mean they have difficulty socialising, or they spend a considerable amount of time on their own. This can have a big impact on their quality of life and sense of wellbeing, so it is important to help service users to maintain their social life and their interests, if this is what they want.

Helping service users to maintain their social life and interests

You may be able to help in the following ways:

- If a service user is unable to leave their home often, help them to stay in touch with the outside world. Talk to them about what you have seen in the local area – for example any changes on their street, new shops that have opened up on the high street, what the neighbours are growing in their gardens and so on. You could also talk about things that are happening in the wider world, for example, the latest news stories.

- Hobbies and interests are an expression of a person's individuality. Encourage service users to take an interest in hobbies or pastimes, if they wish. This may not be part of your job description, but you may have time during your visits to talk to them about their interests, past and present. The person may enjoy talking about something that they have knowledge and expertise about. It will also enable you to investigate the possibility of the person continuing their hobby if they would like to.

- Talk to your supervisor about ways to enable the service user to have more social opportunities.

- Find out about different social activities in the area so that you can let service users know about them. By providing them with information, you are enabling them to make choices.

- Be aware of services that are available to people at home, such as:

  - talking books and talking newspapers

  - mobile library services

  - television and radio programmes

  - befriending services (some organisations offer telephone befriending services as well as home visits)

  - faith groups, ministers or local religious leaders can often be helpful in arranging 'spiritual' support and a link with a person's religious or cultural heritage and community

  - distance learning programmes

  - internet-based activities, such as online discussion forums and e-learning courses

- Be aware that special occasions (such as birthdays) or religious or cultural holidays can be difficult times for people who are lonely or apart from their families, friends or social group.

- Talk to service users about the holidays and occasions that are important to them, and the memories and associations they have and whether there are particular celebrations or religious practices that are important to them.

Transport

If you are arranging transport for a service user you will need to make sure that it is accessible/appropriate for them.

Most public buildings and venues will be wheelchair accessible, but it is worth finding out about access to make sure a service user will be able to get into and around a building.

If you use your own car to assist service users to go shopping or to leave their home, you must be correctly insured. Talk to your supervisor and motor insurer to make sure you have the right cover.

Culture and religion

'Culture' can be described as the habits, customs, attitudes and way of life we absorb from our environment. Our cultural influences include a combination of nationality, religion, language, family traditions, politics and history. During your work you are likely to come into contact with service users from many different cultures. The extent to which a person maintains their original culture or adopts elements of the culture in which they now live will vary according to each individual.

When working with service users:

- Don't make assumptions based on your first impressions of a person.

- Comply with the ground rules of a service user's household.

- Take an interest in cultural backgrounds different from your own.

- Observe the service user's way of life, routines and customs. Ask questions in a sensitive and respectful way and be willing to talk about your own culture so that both you and the service user find out what you have in common, as well as any differences.

Be aware of:

- People who may practice many, few, none or all of the religious and cultural practices they inherited. Others may have converted to another religion during their lifetime.

- People who may have strong opinions (either positive or negative) about their religion and that of others.

- Different rules about diet. For example, Jewish people and Muslims don't eat pork, Hindus don't eat beef and Muslims and people from some branches of Christianity may not drink alcohol. Some religions also have special food preparation practices, such as Kosher (Jewish) and Halal (Muslim). The extent to which people follow these rules will vary.

- Special clothing. For example Sikh men may wear a turban, and many Muslim women wear headscarves to cover their hair and wear modest clothing.

- Religious customs such as saying grace before meals and the Jewish observance of the Sabbath (a weekly day of worship and rest which runs from Friday evening to Saturday evening).

- Courtesies and customs relating to house visits. For example in a Muslim household you may be asked to remove your shoes before entering the house.

- Different ceremonies that mark key stages in people's lives, such as birth, puberty, marriage and death.

- Different interpretations of body language or hand signals. Some gestures you commonly use may mean something else to a person from another culture.

- Special festivals, eg Easter, Jewish New Year, Orthodox festivals, the Atonement, Diwali.

- The language that service users speak. It may be appropriate to learn some words from their language.

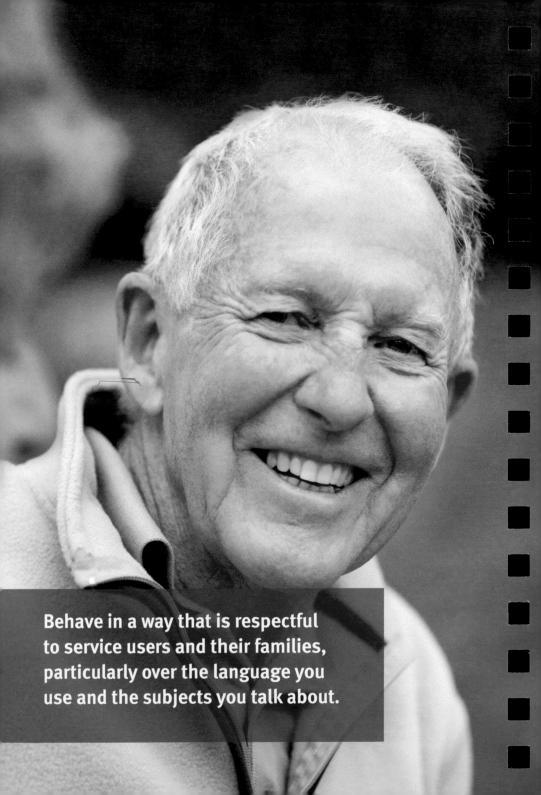

Behave in a way that is respectful
to service users and their families,
particularly over the language you
use and the subjects you talk about.

19   Self-expression and sexuality

Sexuality is a fundamental part of people's lives and plays a big part in how we see ourselves. We express our sexual identity in all sorts of ways, such as how we dress and how we interact with other people, and our friends and family relationships.

It is important to recognise that service users have their own sense of their sexual identity and their own set of attitudes and values relating to sex. It is important to be tolerant of others' views and lifestyles. Never discriminate against a service user on the basis of their sexual orientation, whether they are married, are in a civil partnership, have other types of relationships or have none at all.

There are various things to take into account when thinking about service users' sexuality.

- Many older service users grew up during a time when attitudes towards sex and sexuality were very different. They may find modern attitudes, for example openness about sex or the acceptance of different sexual orientations, difficult to come to terms with.

- A service user's personality, as well as their background, can affect whether or not they are open about sexual matters.

- Some service users may not wish to discuss matters relating to sex, their sexuality or personal relationships because they fear disapproval or prejudice from others.

- Society plays an important part in how people perceive sex and sexuality. Often the sexuality of older people and those who are disabled or ill is overlooked.

- Looking and feeling attractive can play a big part in people's sense of self-esteem.

- Health conditions and disabilities may affect people's sexual health and prevent sexual activity. This can have an impact on their general wellbeing.

- Sexual desire is not necessarily affected by age. However, the physical aspects of ageing may have a negative effect people's sex lives.

Maintaining boundaries

- Maintain appropriate professional relationships with service users. This means respecting their privacy about their sexuality and relationships.

- Behave in a way that is respectful to service users and their families, particularly over the language you use and the subjects you talk about.

- Services users are often interested in the people who provide their care, and may sometimes ask questions about your family relationships. Be cautious about how much information you share and do not divulge any information which you would rather keep private.

- Be clear that you will not take part in jokes or conversation of a sexual nature if they become offensive to you, or others.

- Occasionally you might find that you become the focus of a service user's attempt to express their sexuality. Discuss this with your supervisor and ask for advice about how to handle the situation if you need it.

- If a service user behaves in a sexually inappropriate way towards you or asks you to be involved in any sexual activity, for example watching adult videos, state firmly but politely that this is something you cannot do. Talk to your supervisor about the situation.

- Humour can be a good way of letting out pent-up feelings and dealing with awkward situations.

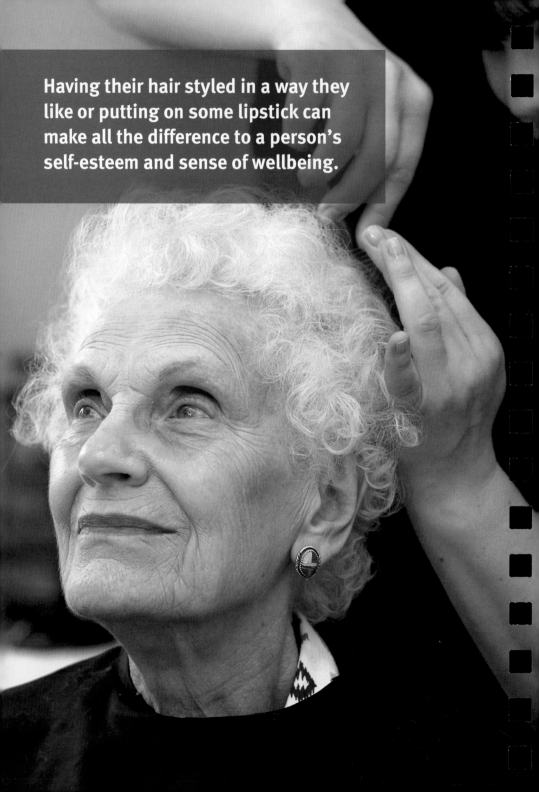

Having their hair styled in a way they like or putting on some lipstick can make all the difference to a person's self-esteem and sense of wellbeing.

20 Washing and dressing

Washing and getting dressed are routines of everyday life, but they are also very personal and intimate tasks. Think about your own daily routines – you probably like to wash your hair in a particular way, or perhaps you always choose your clothes and lay them out before having a shower. Your service user will also have their own way of doing things, so it is important to find out about their preferences, make sure they are comfortable and ensure their privacy and dignity are respected.

Always remember the principles of good practice when you are helping a person to wash or get dressed (see *Chapter 1 – Principles of good care practice*):

- **Communication:** make sure there is good two-way communication so that your service users' rights and choices are always respected.

- **Dignity:** do everything you can to make sure your service users don't feel embarrassed or undignified, or that their privacy has not been invaded.

- **Confidentiality:** information about your service users should only be shared when necessary, in accordance with your organisation's guidelines.

- **Anti-discriminatory practice:** take care not to treat any client differently because of who they are or the way they choose to live.

When you are helping someone to wash and dress, you should also bear in mind health and safety issues (see *Chapter 5 – Health and safety at work*) and techniques for moving and handling (see *Chapter 6 – Helping service users to move*).

Different approaches for different people

Your service users are individuals with different needs and preferences, so it is not possible to describe exactly what to do in every situation. They (and their families) will help you to work out the best way of doing things. This should be described in their care plans, however you should also ask the service user's preferences if you are unsure.

This chapter gives some general points that will apply in all situations, as well as a few points that are specific to certain activities. There is also a checklist to help you plan and carry out different tasks.

General guidance

- Prepare for the task ahead. If you need to put equipment in place or move furniture out of the way, check first with your service user and seek their agreement. Remember where things belong so that you can put these items back afterwards.

- Make sure that you are ready yourself. Do you need to wash your hands? What guidance has your agency given you? Is your hair tied back? Have you put on any protective clothing, such as an apron or gloves? Have you removed any jewellery that could be a hazard to you or others?

- As you go along, check that your service user is comfortable and happy with what you are doing.

- Wherever possible, encourage your service user to carry out any tasks that they can do for themselves, even if it takes them more time than it would if you did it for them.

- When you have finished, clear up. Dry up any spilled water, move furniture back to its original place, hang wet towels where they can dry and dispose of any rubbish. Make sure that your service user can reach any items they may need later. Always put things back where they belong, and leave your service user's home in a state that they are happy with.

Bathing and washing

Bathing and washing are usually private, personal tasks, and your client might feel embarrassed about being undressed in front of you. Do all you can to protect their privacy and dignity.

- Be sensitive to the service user's feeling of embarrassment about being undressed or having to be assisted with intimate personal care.

- Make sure curtains or blinds are closed if necessary.

- Cover up any undressed part of the person's body when you are not in the process of washing that particular part.

- When helping someone use the shower or bath, limit the time they are undressed to a minimum.

- Remember that children, older people, those with reduced mental capacity or mobility, or skin sensitivities or sensory impairment will all be more vulnerable to the risk of scalding.

- Consider the type of bath taps, including mixer taps, or type of shower to be used. Occupational therapists can give advice on suitable adaptive equipment if, for example, a thermostatic mixing valve is needed for safety purposes.

- Run cold water into the bath before adding hot water; mix the water thoroughly and check the temperature at both ends of the bath.

- A risk assessment should determine the appropriate water temperature for the service user. Water temperature must not exceed 44°C for bathing or 41°C for showering.

- Your employer should have a policy on how to check water temperature. The immersible variety of thermometer may be more reliable for baths than the float-on type. Taking the temperature of a shower is substantially less reliable than a bath. Bath scoop thermometers may be used in showers to take the temperature of water close to the shower head.

- Help the service user into the bath.

- Never add hot water to a bath when the service user is already in it.

- Skin must be properly dry before dressing to ensure the person does not get cold and that their skin does not become sore.

- Pay particular attention to drying feet, the groin and genitals, buttocks, under arms and under women's breasts, ensuring this is done thoroughly.

- Use talcum powder sparingly if the person uses it, and apply deodorant to dry skin only. Used incorrectly, both talc and deodorant can irritate the skin.

- Safety in bathrooms is important because of the risks of slips on wet surfaces. Keep bathrooms tidy and mop up spills before they become a hazard.

Helping a service user to get dressed

When helping a service user with their clothes, you may have little choice about dressing techniques. However, the following ideas may be helpful.

- Always think about the service user's privacy and dignity. If necessary, draw curtains or blinds.

- It is easiest to put socks on first, then trousers, then shoes.

- Encourage service users to wear shoes rather than slippers. Shoes offer better support for people's feet, and people often walk with a shuffle in slippers which means they are more likely to trip.

- Make sure that the service user's circulation isn't restricted by shoelaces that are tied too tight, the elastic tops of stockings or socks, or elastic cuffs.

- With non-opening items of clothing, such as dresses or T-shirts, help the person to put their arms through the sleeves first, then gather the back of the garment with your hands and take the garment over the person's head.

- If your service user is unable to stand, it is easier to help them put on pants and trousers when they are lying down rather than sitting up.

- If it is difficult to help a service user put on tights, elastic-topped stockings could be an easier option. If the person wears suspenders, make sure they are not sitting on them in discomfort.

Appearance and grooming

For many people, the way they look has a big effect on the way they feel about themselves. Having their hair styled in a way they like or putting on some lipstick can make all the difference to a person's self-esteem and sense of wellbeing. When you are helping a service user with their personal grooming, remember the following:

- Brush or comb a service user's hair from the roots. If their hair is tangled, put gentle pressure on the top of their head with one hand while combing or brushing with the other, so that you don't pull at the roots of the hair.

- Don't assume that a service user with little hair doesn't want to have it combed or brushed. The scalp will benefit from the stimulation.

- When using hairpins and grips, take care not to scratch your service user's scalp or pull their hair.

- If you need to rub lotion into a service user's scalp, do it gently, with the tips of the fingers.

- Be very careful when cutting a person's fingernails – gentle filing or nail clippers may be preferable to using scissors. Your organisation may have their own policy regarding this or there may be a risk assessment for your client that outlines procedures to be followed.

- You should avoid cutting or clipping toenails, because of the risk of accidentally cutting the service user's skin, as this could lead to an infection or gangrene. If your client's toenails or feet need attention, make a note of this and report it so that a visit from a chiropodist can be arranged.

- Your agency may have policies and procedures relating to cutting people's hair and shaving men's faces. (Typically an agency may state that shaving should only be done with an electric razor).

For people who are in bed

If you are carrying out washing, dressing or grooming tasks with a person who is in bed, extra care is needed when handling water, especially hot water. Non-slip mats are useful to keep bowls stable (see *Chapter 23 – Aids and adaptations*). It is also a good idea to have some towels close to hand in case of spills.

Washing and dressing checklist

	Things to consider	What you will need
Bathing/ washing	Doors Draughts Space Water temperature Spilled water	Towels Wash cloths Soap Laundry basket Non-slip mat Shower/bath seat
Dressing	Going out? Having visitors? Temperature	Service user's choice of clothes Long-handled zipper Stocking or sock gutter Shoe horn Mirror
Appearance	Activities and plan for the day	Mirror Brush and comb Jewellery/watch Make up
Hair washing	Spilled water Water temperature Draughts	Service user's choice of shampoo and conditioner Towels Brushes/combs/hairdryer
Going to the toilet	Ensure space Prepare room Protect bed/chairs etc	Container for soiled pads Toilet paper or wash cloths Pads, pants Commode chair/bedpan/bottle
Shaving	Towels for protection Spilled water	Hot water Non-slip mats for water container Razor, brushes, shaving soap etc Towels Dry hands for electric plugs for electric razor
Teeth cleaning	Towels for protection	Toothpaste/powder Denture dish Denture fluid Floss Rinsing water

Things to look out for
Red skin, especially in the skin folds Breaks in the skin Abnormality with nose, ears, eyes Prostheses (false limbs or body parts that need to be removed) Areas service user cannot reach
Wrinkles in clothes Sitting on suspenders Ease or difficulty of dressing Pains, discomfort Shoulders and crotch comfortable
Enjoyment of brushing/combing Dandruff Nail care – clean/smooth
Check behind ears Check scalp Brush dandruff from shoulders
Red marks on skin Urine/faeces condition Wash hands – both service user and careworker
Parts not reached by service user Cuts Skin condition
Damaged gums Ill-fitting dentures Pain Halitosis Sore/cracked lips

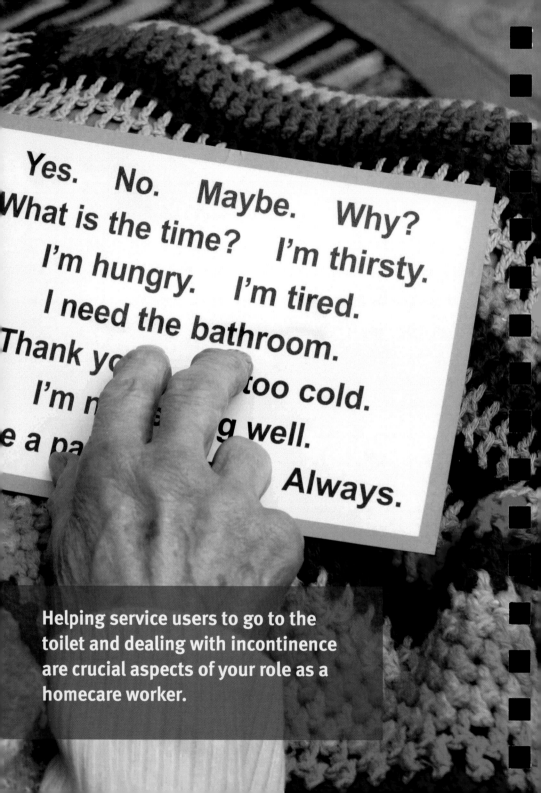

Yes.   No.   Maybe.   Why?
What is the time?   I'm thirsty.
I'm hungry.   I'm tired.
I need the bathroom.
Thank yo...   ...too cold.
I'm n...   ...g well.
e a pa...   ...Always.

Helping service users to go to the
toilet and dealing with incontinence
are crucial aspects of your role as a
homecare worker.

21   Continence and using the toilet

Helping service users to go to the toilet and dealing with incontinence are crucial aspects of your role as a homecare worker. It is an area where you need to be particularly sensitive and consider service users' dignity at all times.

What is incontinence?

Incontinence is a term that describes the accidental or involuntary loss of urine from the bladder (urinary incontinence) or faeces from the bowel (faecal or bowel incontinence). It is a widespread condition that can range from an occasional 'leak' to complete loss of bladder or bowel control.

Incontinence usually affects older people, but is not an inevitable part of the ageing process. It can sometimes be cured, but where this is not the case it can be managed through a range of methods. This chapter outlines some of the causes of incontinence, and ways of supporting service users to manage it.

Understanding service users' needs

Remember that a service user who has continence problems may feel embarrassed or ashamed, so you need to do everything you can to preserve their dignity and maintain their sense of self-esteem. Your approach will depend on the person and your relationship with them.

Whatever the situation, give the service user as much privacy as possible. Never say anything that may make them feel as though you are 'telling them off', or that makes them feel careless or stupid, or increases their embarrassment.

It is vital to:

- **Show sensitivity** – imagine how service users might feel and be sensitive to their needs and feelings.

- **Be aware of your responsibilities.** Are you familiar with your agency's policies? Are you clear about your own job description? If your observations of a service user give you any cause for concern, talk to your supervisor.

Incontinence can also have a big impact on a service user's family members. You may find that you have an important role in explaining facts, listening to problems and helping service users and their families come to terms with what can be a difficult situation.

If you notice signs of incontinence

You may work with service users who have already had their continence needs assessed, in which case you will follow the care plan that has been agreed with them.

However, you may be the first person to be aware that a service user has begun to have continence problems. They may be reluctant to talk to you about it, and may deny or hide what is happening. Hopefully you will be able to gain their confidence and, with sensitivity, find out what the problems are so that you can let your supervisor know. However, if you have concerns and a service user won't discuss any problem, you should report your observations so that the situation can be monitored and the service user's needs met.

With the service user's agreement, your agency can refer them to a practice nurse, community nurse or continence service for a full assessment. A care plan is then agreed with the service user and regularly reviewed.

Types of incontinence

Urinary incontinence

Urinary incontinence can occur for several reasons.

- Functional incontinence – This happens when a service user can't get to the toilet in time. It is the most common cause of incontinence among older people and can occur for various reasons. The service user might have trouble getting out of a chair quickly, for example, or might be unable to get out of bed easily at night. They might be unable to undo zips or buttons.

- Urge incontinence – When someone gets an unpredictable and sudden urge to go to the toilet. It is caused by overactive bladder muscles, which mean the sphincter cannot withstand the pressure behind it. This can be caused by an infection. A service user may feel as if they want to go to the toilet frequently, even though there is not very much urine in their bladder.

- Reflex incontinence – Usually, a person knows that they need to go to the toilet because the bladder sends a message to the brain. In reflex incontinence, the message doesn't get through, so the bladder empties without warning. This can be caused by damage to the nervous system, for example because of an injury to the spine. It can also happen when someone is very frightened.

- Overflow incontinence – When urine 'dribbles out', either because the muscles (or sphincter) that control the release of urine from the bladder do not work as well as they should, or because urine is being held in the bladder (urine retention) due to pressure from an enlarged prostate gland. There is a danger of infection in the retained urine, so this condition needs careful treatment. If you notice that a service user is showing signs of overflow incontinence, report it to your supervisor.

- Stress incontinence – This happens when the bladder muscles contract suddenly without warning. It can occur when a person sneezes, coughs or laughs, and is likely to affect women more than men.

Other factors may aggravate urinary incontinence:

- Coffee or other drinks containing caffeine make the bladder contract more frequently.

- Diuretics – drugs which encourage the body to excrete urine.

- Alcohol, which acts like a diuretic.

- Painkillers (analgesics) can slow down the messages being sent from the bladder to the brain.

- A lack of routine for going to the toilet can lead to random occurrences of incontinence.

- Constipation can mean extra pressure is put on the bladder.

- Fear of incontinence. It is normal for adults to drink about 10 cupfuls of liquid in 24 hours and most people have their own personal, daily routine for going to the toilet. Someone who is afraid of being incontinent may cut down on the amount of liquid they drink. This may lead to a urinary infection which can cause further incontinence. Cutting back on liquid intake also increases the risk of dehydration.

- Service users who experience incontinence may go to extreme lengths to hide this fact, although it is very difficult to hide because odours, stains or a change in the person's habits may be obvious. If the person gets an infection because of an untreated urinary problem, this can increase the chance of further incontinence problems.

Faecal incontinence

The causes of faecal incontinence are similar to those of urinary incontinence, for example weakened muscles, an unsuitable diet and the inability to get to the toilet in time. It is probably less common than urinary incontinence but can be more distressing.

The best way for someone to maintain regular bowel movements is to:

- Drink plenty of liquids, especially a hot drink with breakfast.

- Eat foods that contain fibre, such as brown bread, cereals and fruit.

- Take appropriate exercise – a short walk, for example.

- Go to the toilet after meals.

Helping service users to use the toilet

Often older people are able to regain continence with the right support. To help them maintain their dignity, self-esteem and quality of life, it is vital to support service users to maintain continence rather than turn to bedpans, special pants or pads as the first option:

- Does the service user have a programme or pattern for using the toilet? If so, can you help them to follow their programme, perhaps with a system of reminders?

- Can the service user get to the toilet as quickly and easily as possible? Is getting out of the chair a problem? Is furniture in the way? Are there obstacles in the bathroom?

- Can the service user undo their clothes easily? Do they have too many layers of clothing to deal with quickly? Could velcro fastenings or larger buttons make it easier? Would someone who uses a wheelchair find back openings helpful?

- Would reminders about the sequence of actions when going to the toilet help the service user?

When helping a client to use toilet facilities

Think ahead – especially about space management:

- Practice moving and handling techniques beforehand.

- Remember that for every service user you will have a different plan of action.

- Ask members of the family for hints on their techniques.

- Try to leave your service users alone when they are using the toilet or bedpan, and shut doors or draw curtains so that they have privacy.

- Would the service user benefit from aids, such as a raised toilet seat or grab rails on the way to the bathroom and in the bathroom itself? If so, you should report this to your supervisor.

- Are toilet paper and any other cleansing aids within the service user's reach?

Continence aids

If the service user is unable to use the toilet, they may need to use one of the following aids:

Urine bottle

These are for male service users. They should be kept somewhere where the service user can easily reach them and put them down again after use. A bottle should always be covered when not in use and emptied as often as possible. A service user may find it easier to use a bottle when sitting on the edge of the bed or standing next to a chair.

Urinals made for women are also available. Some service users may find them easier to use than a bedpan.

Bedpan

Ask service users how you can best help them to use a bedpan. Some people lie on one side and roll back onto the pan. If the head of the bed can be raised, the service user may find it easier to use the bedpan in a more upright position. The bedpan can also be used in a sitting position, in which case the person may find it more comfortable if they bend their knees.

Pads and incontinence pants

A nurse or continence adviser should give advice on the best type of pads or pants for a service user.

There are also more invasive aids that you may come across such as a catheter (a tube inserted into the body to drain urine) or a stoma (an artificial opening in the person's abdomen). If you are required to assist with these you will be given specialist training.

It is important for a service user who uses pads to be washed (or helped to wash) between their legs frequently. The skin must be dried thoroughly afterwards.

Waterproof bedding

Plastic or rubber sheeting can be used to protect the bed. A draw sheet can also be used. This is a narrow sheet that goes across the bed under a service user's lower back and thighs, that can be removed easily if it gets wet. It should also be checked for wrinkles which could cause discomfort to the service user.

Supporting someone who uses a wheelchair

If a service user who uses a wheelchair has continence problems, wipe the seat of the chair regularly and make sure the cushion covers are washed often. Also check the cushion filling in case the material begins to break down.

Spotting potential health problems

The waste produced by our bodies can give clues about how well the body is functioning. Urine should be a pale yellow colour with only a slight smell.

Let your supervisor know if you notice, or if a service user tells you about, any of the following:

- Very dark urine (this could be caused by eating certain foods, but it is also a sign of dehydration or illness).

- Urine with a strong smell.

- Cloudy urine.

- Pain or a stinging feeling when passing urine.

- Difficulty in passing any urine, or only passing tiny amounts.

Observations of service users' stools (faeces) can also be important. Stools should be dark brown and formed, but not hard. If stools are yellow or very liquid (ie the service user has diarrhoea), or if they contain undigested food, you should report this. If a service user's stools are black, this may be because they are taking iron supplements.

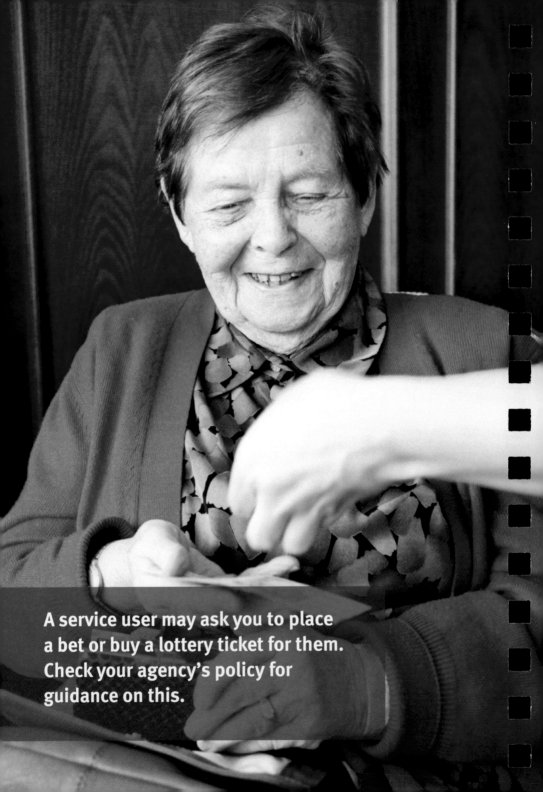

A service user may ask you to place a bet or buy a lottery ticket for them. Check your agency's policy for guidance on this.

22 Household tasks and money management

Many service users like to have a clean and well run home, with domestic chores done efficiently and in a timely manner. Some degree of order is important if a service user is in receipt of homecare. For example, there needs to be food in the fridge for the careworker to prepare, and clean towels available for the service user's bath. Some service users also regard a clean and orderly house as essential for their self-esteem, while others regard it as less important.

Your role may involve carrying out household tasks on a service user's behalf, because they cannot manage them for themselves or prefer to devote their energies to other tasks. As far as possible, you should enable the service user to make their own choices and, where they want to, get involved in tasks. Encourage them to make their own decisions about what they would like to buy or how they would like you to do things.

When it comes to handling money, it is essential to follow the procedures laid down by your agency. They are there to safeguard the interests of service users and to protect you.

Money matters

Make sure you are clear about the agreement that the service user (or their family members) made with your agency about money matters. The following section gives some general points on money-related tasks; refer to your agency's policies for specific guidance relating to your role.

- There should be a system in place to record any transactions, such as shopping, that you carry out on a service user's behalf. Usually the service user will confirm each transaction by signing the record. Follow your agency's procedures for this and make sure the records are kept up to date.

- Always check that you have been given the right amount of money before you leave a bank or post office, and that you have been given the correct change before you leave a shop.

- If you pay a bill over the counter on a service user's behalf, make sure it is stamped as paid and make a record of the payment in the appropriate way.

- Follow your agency's advice about withdrawing cash from service users' accounts. Make sure you carry any required ID and authorisation when making a withdrawal. Seek guidance from your agency about the safekeeping of cashpoint cards and PIN numbers and what to do if they are lost.

- If you are asked to deposit money in the bank for a service user, follow your agency's guidance about how to record this. You will probably need to obtain evidence of the transaction from the bank and make a record of the deposit that is then signed off by the service user.

- Your agency may have special procedures to safeguard careworkers who regularly deposit or collect money or other valuables, for example by making sure they vary their routes or schedules. Make sure you follow these procedures if they apply to you.

- Your role may include helping service users with their budgeting. This might involve advising on the allocation of weekly income to pay bills, buy shopping and make other regular payments. Do not give advice about financial matters that are outside your remit, such as savings or investment advice. Instead, let the service user know that they should talk to someone with the appropriate experience and qualifications, who is authorised to give such advice.

- A service user may ask you to place a bet or buy a lottery ticket for them. Check your agency's policy for guidance on this.

- If you notice that a service user is finding it more difficult to manage their money, let your supervisor know.

Maintaining professional boundaries

Remember that, while you may get on well with service users, you should always keep your relationship with them on a professional footing. This includes avoiding any personal financial arrangements with a service user. For example, it would not be acceptable to borrow money from, or lend money to, a service user or their family.

- Follow your agency's policy on gifts between careworkers and service users. Usually careworkers are required to politely refuse gifts, or only accept gifts of low monetary value (see *Chapter 4 – Service users and their homes*).

- Never accept a loan from, or lend money to, a service user.

- Careworkers should not sell anything to or buy anything from a service user.

- Don't get involved in the making or witnessing of a service user's will or any other legal matters.

- Never try to involve a service user in any sort of lottery or gambling syndicate.

- Careworkers should not gain personally from purchases they make on behalf of service users, for example two-for-one offers or loyalty card points.

Shopping

Shopping list – Encourage service users to make their own shopping lists. If they have trouble writing, make a list with tick boxes. Encourage other visitors to the home to make a note if things like sugar or toilet paper are getting low, so that they can be replaced. Go through the list carefully with the service user, and don't assume that they will always want the same things.

Choice – If a service user is able to go out, and there is enough time, encourage them to go with you to the shops. This will provide an outing and enable them to make choices about what to buy. (You will need to check the risk assessment for accompanying the service user out of the home, or arrange for one to be carried out). If they can't go with you or do not wish to, suggest things that they might like to purchase. When making the list try to give the service user an idea of the shop and what might be on display, what's new and what's on special offer. If they have seen something advertised on television, ask if they would like to try it. Small one-portion packs may be a good way for a person to try something new.

Quantities – If you do the shopping regularly you will have a good idea of the quantities a service user needs, but always check what size of packets, for example, they want. Buying large packets might mean food goes to waste if the service user can't use it quickly enough.

Cost – People who cannot shop for themselves can easily lose track of what things cost. Try to help service users stay in touch with prices. Remember that what you think the service user can afford might not be the same as what they would like to pay. They might be able to afford the highest quality products but still prefer to buy the budget brands.

Which shop? – Again, ask the service user what they prefer and use the shop they choose (unless you have instructions as part of a contract).

Payment – Follow your agency's policy about handling money and agree with the service user how you will pay for the shopping. Encourage the service user to do as much as possible, for example checking receipts. Make sure any records are kept of what you spend, as outlined above.

Putting shopping away – Suggest that you check through the shopping with the service user when you get home. This is an opportunity to help them keep in touch with prices and the goods on offer. Put things away where the service user would like them and can reach them. If it helps the service user, open packaging that they might otherwise find difficult, such as milk bottle lids, cartons or jars.

Cleaning

Cleaning materials – Many household cleaning products contain toxic or harmful substances, so take care when using and storing them, particularly in the home of a service user who has vision problems (see *Chapter 8 – The human body and health*).

Waste bins – Empty bins regularly and throw away rubbish in sealed bags. Follow your agency guidelines for the disposal of incontinence pads and medical waste.

Sinks, basins and baths – These should always be cleaned after use. Remove any hair from the plughole, wipe taps and make sure the soap dish is clean.

Floors – Mop bathroom, toilet or kitchen floors dry after you have cleaned them. Dry carpeted floors if they get wet, and vacuum regularly. Make sure mats or carpets are secured so that they don't cause accidents.

Surfaces – Keep furniture surfaces dust-free. If a service user has asthma, wipe surfaces with a damp cloth. Picture frames and mirrors, which collect dust along the top edges, should also be damp-dusted.

Armchairs – Give the cushions a shake and check to see whether anything has fallen down the sides of the cushions.

Ironing – Ask service users how they like their ironing to be done. When you are finished, unplug the iron and leave it in a safe place, especially if it is still hot. Allow ironed clothes to air before putting them away.

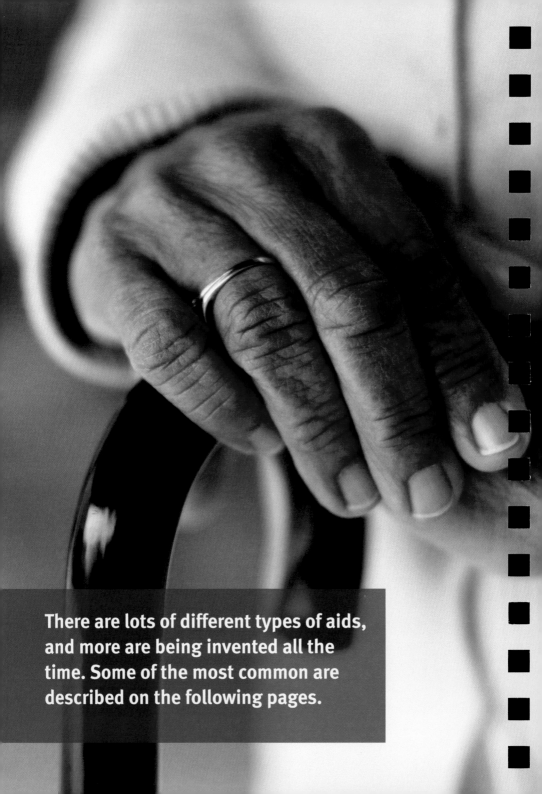

There are lots of different types of aids, and more are being invented all the time. Some of the most common are described on the following pages.

23   Aids and adaptations

There are numerous aids and adaptations that can help service users to remain independent and carry out tasks for themselves. It is not possible to cover them all in detail here, so this chapter:

- Suggests when an aid might be helpful.

- Describes the most commonly used aids.

- Lets you know where you can find out more about aids, or source the aids yourself.

The experts on aids and adaptations are occupational therapists (see *Chapter 24 – The social care team,* for more information about their role). However, your day-to-day contact with service users means you are likely to notice when aids and adaptations could become helpful. If you know what is available you will be able to make informed suggestions either to service users and their families or to your agency.

When is an aid or adaptation helpful?

You might think that it is best to suggest an aid as soon as you see that a service user is finding an everyday task difficult. However this may not always be the case. In some circumstances, making an effort to carry out a task can:

- Exercise a person's muscles, help their blood circulation and help to keep joints and skin supple.

- Create a sense of satisfaction and achievement for a service user and maintain a sense of 'normality'.

However, if any of the following occurs, it is time to think about aids and adaptations:

- A service user begins to have accidents, for example dropping or breaking objects, because their eyesight is poor or their grip has become weak.

- A service user cannot deal with these kinds of accidents because of old age, a health condition or injury. For example, a person may not need an aid because they occasionally drop things, but they may need an aid to help pick them up again.

- A task causes continuing frustration or pain for a service user.

- A service user begins to have accidents, or is at risk of injuring themselves – for example they burn themselves because they can no longer lift the kettle easily.

- A service user's personal appearance and dignity begin to suffer.

What sorts of aids are available?

There are lots of different types of aids, and more are being invented all the time. Some of the most common are illustrated and described on the following pages.

Remember, aids don't have to be custom-made. Everyday household items such as pegs or a tall stool can be used to help a service user to perform a task.

It is also worth bearing in mind that an aid is only an aid if it suits the individual service user – otherwise it is likely to cause problems of its own.

Aids for general use

Helping hand – This is a 'stick' about 18 inches (45 centimetres) long with a squeezable handle at one end and a sprung gripper at the other. It helps a service user to reach further or grasp things that they might find difficult to hold with their fingers. For example, a service user might use it to pull curtains that they would otherwise not be able to reach. The weight a helping hand can take will depend on how tightly the service user can grip the handle.

Grippers – These help service users with a weak grip to unscrew jars or bottles. They look a bit like a pair of scissors but, instead of blades, they come with rings of different sizes that fit over a container lid. Another useful type of gripper is the sort that looks like a thin rubber mat, which can be used to hold slippery containers or get a good grip on a lid.

Non-slip mat – Flexible, rubbery mats that create a non-slip surface, for example to prevent a plate and cup from sliding on a tray. They come in different sizes and shapes and can be very useful for all sorts of items in the home, such as a service user's tooth mug, writing pad, mixing bowl or telephone.

Pegs – There are many uses for pegs, for example holding clothes, curtains or sheets out of the way, stopping the pages of a book from turning over or attaching messages in visible places. Colourful pegs of different sizes can be bought, but ordinary clothes pegs are a cheaper alternative and are just as effective.

Electrical plugs with handles – These enable a service user who has trouble gripping things to plug and unplug electrical appliances.

Portable doorbell amplifier – An amplifier, installed by a electrician, that a service user can carry to any part of the house or even the garden so that they can hear the doorbell.

Rubber fingers/rubber thimbles – These are normally used in offices for leafing through paper documents, but they can also be useful in the home, for example when turning the pages of a book or opening plastic bags.

Sheepskin – Real sheepskin or sheepskin-like fabric can have many uses. It can make a chair more comfortable to sit on, provide warmth and comfort for hands or feet, and be used as an armrest or as padding for heels or other joints where pressure might occur.

Sliding board – This is a well-polished board of about 12 inches (30 cm) in width and 24 inches (60cm) in length, with well-rounded, smooth corners. It is used to help a person move from, for example, a chair to a bed.

Tall stools – Stools can be placed at strategic points in the home so that a service user can have a rest when going from room to room, for example, or take the weight off their feet while cooking or washing.

Transfer sling – A rectangular aid made of slightly flexible material, about three feet in length and a foot wide, with handles at each end. It enables a careworker to support a service user's back and hold the service user in a particular position when helping them move from one position to another.

Trolley or mobile tray – Trays with wheels that can help a wheelchair user to carry things, or that provide support to help a service user walk as well as move things from place to place.

Walking stick – A service user should use a walking stick on their 'bad' side so that it takes the pressure off their weak, injured or painful leg or foot. A walking stick should have a rubber stopper on the end so that it doesn't slip.

Aids for the kitchen

Gas cooker controls – Special Braille controls can be installed for service users with sight problems. The service user's gas company will have a department that deals with adaptations to gas appliances.

Kettle and jug tipper – This is a frame, made of wood or plastic, into which a jug or kettle fits. It helps a service user to tip liquids from one container to another.

Long-handled or enlarged tap fittings – These are useful in the kitchen and the bathroom. Some types can be clipped over existing taps and do not need special plumbing.

Aids for the bedroom

Urine bottles – For a male service user who finds it hard to get around or to get in and out of bed at night, a urine bottle is invaluable. It can be carried around easily and discreetly, and a bottle with a stopper can be used on journeys and outings, especially if there is any doubt about the availability of toilets.

Dressing stick – This is a stick, which can be straight or curved, with a hook or rubber finger at one end. It can help a service user who has restricted movement to open the sleeve or leg of a garment, pull up straps or lift clothes on to their shoulders, for example. Service users will develop their own techniques for using a dressing stick, depending on their abilities.

Eye-level clothes rails – A rail can be used to hang clothes at a height that a service user can reach more easily. This can be particularly helpful for a person who uses a wheelchair.

Stocking or sock gutter – This is a curved sheet of plastic with two long tapes attached to either side. The service user gathers the sock or stocking and puts it over one end of the plastic 'gutter', and then puts it on the floor and puts their foot in the open end. They then pull the gutter up using the tapes, bringing the sock or stocking with it.

Zip hook or button hook – A stick with a hook or loop of metal at the end, it enables a service user to pull up the tag of a zip or pull a button through a button hole.

Aids for the bathroom

Mirrors – A mobile, hinged, or retractable mirror can be helpful if a service user can no longer see into their bathroom mirror.

Raised toilet seats – These can be fixed permanently to a toilet seat or taken on and off according to use. There are also many kinds of commodes, commode wheelchairs and special toilet seats.

Suction mats – These can vary in size from small mats for a bar of soap to larger ones that can be placed in the bath to prevent a service user from slipping.

Thick toothbrush handles – Useful for a service user who has trouble gripping things. Thick-handled cutlery, pens and pencils can also be useful.

Toothpaste dispenser – A small device, fixed to the wall at a suitable level, which enables a service user to put toothpaste on their brush using only one hand.

Aids for the living room

Book holder/stand and page-turner – A slanting wooden or plastic frame on a horizontal 'foot' that supports a book for a service user who is unable to hold one. Some come with page-turners, or a stick with a rubber end can be used to turn pages.

Computers and electronic equipment – There are many ways in which computers can help people who are living with a disability or are unable to leave their home. A wide range of electronic gadgets, such as voice-controlled lights, can also be fitted to enable service users with little movement to control their own environment. The occupational therapist can advise on these.

Remote control – A service user who has problems with their sight may find it helpful if you add labels to their existing remote control. Remote controls with large buttons are also available. Remember to leave remote controls in a place where the service user can reach them – a non-slip mat can help to stop them sliding away. For push-button controls on appliances, the service user could use a stick with a rubber finger on the end to press the controls. Make sure that the appliance is stable and will not move or fall when the buttons are pressed.

Telephone receiver stand – A stand for the telephone receiver/handset which means the service user doesn't have to hold the phone during a conversation. An alternative to this could be a phone with a loudspeaker, which can be used without lifting the handset.

Trays – A tray with a bean bag underneath will mould to the shape of the service user's lap to make a secure surface.

Telecare

The term "telecare" is used to describe remote monitoring and communication services that support people to live at home, for example: a sensor under a doormat that alerts a monitoring centre, if a person with dementia leaves the house in the night.

Telecare includes a wide and expanding range of services. Services in this category may also sometimes be known as "tele-health", "e-medication" or other similar names.

Finding out more

- Occupational Therapy departments in hospitals and social services. The service user's GP will have names and contact details.

- Voluntary organisations.

- Specialist shops.

- Aids and adaptations catalogues.

- High street shops such as chemists, department stores and supermarkets, which stock many useful gadgets for the home.

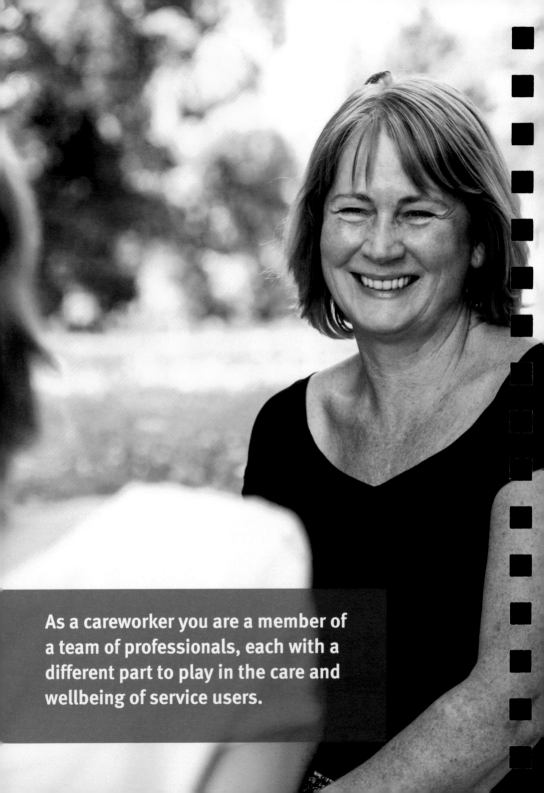

As a careworker you are a member of a team of professionals, each with a different part to play in the care and wellbeing of service users.

24   The social care team

As a careworker you are a member of a team of professionals, each with a different part to play in the care and well-being of service users. This chapter describes the role of some of the professionals that could be members of a service user's care team.

It is important to have a general understanding of the services different team members provide. You should also know which professionals are members of the care team for each service user you work with. This will vary depending on the health and care needs of each individual.

You may not have direct contact with other members of the team, but their recommendations may influence the way you work with service users. In turn, your observations about service users may result in them being referred to one of the specialists described here.

Cooperation and communication between everyone in a person's care team is very important. Always make sure you:

- Support the work of other team members, for example by carrying out instructions or following up treatment or exercise programmes set by another member of the team.

- Report any changes in a service user's health or well-being to your supervisor or to the relevant professional, depending on your agency's guidelines.

- Recognise when you have reached the limits of your own knowledge and let your agency know if you think a service user needs specialist help.

Remember that family carers may be a vital part of a service user's care team. Service users may also be visited by friends, family or by a befriender from a voluntary organisation, for example.

Many of the professionals described here will be employed by the NHS or local authority. Some will work at a day centre, surgery or hospital, while others will visit service users at home.

Audiologist

Audiologists are experts in issues relating to people's ears, hearing and balance. A service user is likely to see an audiologist if they need a hearing aid.

Chiropodist

A chiropodist (or podiatrist) diagnoses and treats foot problems. As well as dealing with common conditions such as fungal infections and corns, they can analyse the way a person walks in order to correct foot problems, help people whose feet have been affected by diseases such as rheumatoid arthritis, and carry out nail surgery using local anaesthetic. Chiropody services can be obtained through health and social services but many people choose to pay privately.

Community or district nurse

Community nurses usually visit service users at home and work within a particular geographical area. Their expertise is in pressure area care, catheters, sterile dressings and the administration of some drugs. They may also undertake manual bowel evacuations and other procedures. Many of these tasks are referred to as 'invasive techniques' and should not usually be carried out by careworkers unless they have had specialist training. Sometimes you may be asked to help, but under the supervision or instruction of the nurse. You may need to follow any instructions or notes made by the nurse in the service user's care plan.

Community psychiatric nurse (CPN)

A CPN is a nurse who supports people with mental health problems, including Alzheimer's disease and other forms of dementia. They usually visit people at home. They may offer practical or emotional support, supervise a service user's medication or injections, and can provide information and advice to help the person's family understand and cope with the illness.

Continence adviser

A continence adviser is a specialist nurse who advises and supports people with bladder and bowel problems or incontinence. They can make home visits to assess a person's needs and advise on treatments, continence aids etc.

Dietitian

A dietitian can assess, diagnose and treat diet and nutrition problems and advise people on how to stay healthy or prevent health problems through their diet. They work with people who have conditions such as diabetes, food allergies, eating disorders, irritable bowel syndrome, heart disease or obesity.

General practitioner (GP) or family doctor

GPs play a key role in a service user's health care. A GP diagnoses diseases or conditions and can prescribe drugs or refer a service user to a specialist service. It is important that the GP is kept informed about any changes you observe in a service user's well-being. A system should be in place to enable this to happen, either via your supervisor or a member of the service user's family.

Health visitor (HV)

Health visitors are registered nurses or midwives with additional training in health and social care matters. Most health visitors work with families to prevent illness and promote the healthy development of babies and young children. Some health visitors are dedicated to the support of older people. They can advise on diet, medication and fall prevention. They can also refer service users to other health and social services and advise on benefits and housing issues.

Occupational therapist (OT)

If a service user is having difficulty carrying out day-to-day tasks, an occupational therapist can offer practical solutions to help them maintain their independence as far as possible. They can advise on aids and devices, as well as therapeutic activities to help maintain or improve movement, coordination or strength. OTs can offer advice on splints and limb supports, and on hobbies and activities that give service users a sense of purpose and achievement. OTs may also assess service users for a wheelchair and help train the service user and their family carers to use it safely.

Optician

Opticians (also known as ophthalmic practitioners or optometrists) test people's vision and check their eye health. They can prescribe glasses and contact lenses, and if necessary, refer a service user to a specialist doctor or eye surgeon for further advice and treatment. Other eye specialists include ophthalmologists, who are trained doctors with specialist knowledge of eye diseases, and orthoptists, who diagnose and treat problems associated with the coordination or movement of the eyes, such as a lazy eye or squint.

240 The social care team

Orthotist and prosthetist

An orthotist advises on medical devices that control or support a part of the body, such as splints or calipers. A prosthetist advises on artificial arms and legs. Both are usually based at a hospital. Services users are likely to be referred to them by a hospital consultant.

Pharmacist

A pharmacist (also called a chemist) ensures that medicines – either prescribed by a GP or bought over the counter – are safely supplied and gives advice on how to take them and any possible side effects. While they can't diagnose illnesses, they can advise on treatments for minor ailments. Some pharmacists set up aids such as managed dosage devices, which contain correct doses of drugs ready for service users. They may also deliver cylinders of oxygen. Pharmacists may offer other services such as blood pressure or cholesterol testing and support to help people manage diabetes or give up smoking.

Physiotherapist

Physiotherapists use movement and exercise to help people with physical problems caused by illness, an accident or ageing. They may give service users exercises to do to help them stay healthy or to improve their movement, or provide manual therapy (where the physiotherapist massages or moves a service user's muscles or limbs). They can advise on wheelchair use, on walking aids, and on sitting or lying positions that will help service users to maintain good posture or avoid pressure sores. They may also visit service users with lung problems to give them treatment to help them breathe or cough. Sometimes the physiotherapist may teach careworkers special exercises for individual service users.

Psychiatrist

Psychiatrists are trained to treat mental illnesses and can prescribe drug treatments for behavioural problems. Psychiatrists and psychologists often work together. An old age psychiatrist, or psychogeriatrician, specialises in the mental health of older people.

Psychologist

Psychologists are experts in human behaviour. They provide a range of treatments or therapies such as group therapy, individual psychotherapy and programmes that help people to modify their behaviour.

Rehabilitation engineer

A rehabilitation engineer is a specialist who advises on and provides mechanical and electronic equipment (known as assistive technology) to help people with physical disabilities live more independently.

Social worker

Social workers tend to specialise in either adult or children's services. Work with adults includes supporting people with mental health problems or learning difficulties and older people. They may help people with problems relating to benefits, housing or health issues. A social worker who works with children and young people may be involved in helping families during a period of crisis and providing support to young people who are leaving care. Social workers often act as case managers, assessing service users' care needs and working with them to put a support plan in place. The social worker's assessment determines the level of financial support the service user receives. These funds may pay for some or all of the service you are providing to the service user, in which case the social worker will monitor the service you are providing through your agency.

Speech and language therapist (SLT)

SLTs are usually employed by the NHS. They are trained to work with people of all ages who have problems with communication, for example because of an injury, neurological condition, cerebral palsy, stroke or learning difficulties. An SLT may also support service users who have problems with chewing or swallowing.

Always remember...

Your role is vital

Giving someone the ability to live at home is one of the most important jobs in the community today. You may be one of a team supporting a person, but as someone who sees service users daily, or almost daily, your contribution to their well-being is vital.

Working in homecare is very demanding, but personally rewarding. By helping service users carry out everyday tasks you can make a big difference to their lives - and give them the greatest gift of all, their independence.

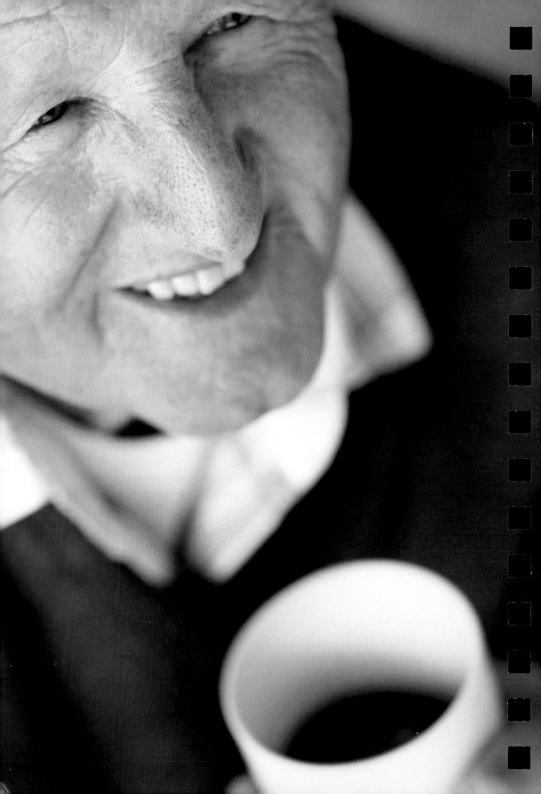

Index

Index

General Practitioner (GP) (general) 64, 65, 91, 98, 148, 156, 165, 233, 240
Giddiness 57
Gifts 27, 220
Glaucoma 85
Good practice 6, 18, 156, 198
Grab rails 213
Grievance 15
Grippers 228
Grooming 203, 204

H
Halal 174, 191
Halitosis (bad breath) 75, 93, 206
Hands
 - *careworkers'* 40, 41, 90, 109, 152, 178, 182, 199, 205, 206
 - *first aid* 60, 61
 - *washing / hygiene* 40, 41, 109, 178, 182, 199, 205, 206
 - *service users'* 73, 74, 82, 99, 116, 152, 185, 192, 229
Hand washing (careworkers) 40, 41, 109, 178, 182, 199
Harmful substances 63, 222
Hazardous substances 32, 35
Hazards in the home 33
Hazards, household 39
Headscarves 191
Health
 - *careworkers'* 14, 15, 47
 - *common conditions* 108-120
 - *emergencies* 57-66
 - *general* 12, 13, 23, 26, 149, 150, 165, 168, 188, 215, 227, 236

 - *human body and health* 70-93
 - *mental health* 18, 96-106, 238
 - *professionals* 148, 236-241
 - *sexual health* 195
 - *smoking* 25, 43, 44, 78, 240
 - *and special diet* 176
Health and safety 15, 32-34, 46, 47, 198
Healthy eating 75, 168, 171, 172, 173, 174, 238
Health visitor 81, 239
Hearing aids 88, 90, 237
Hearing loss 88
Heart (general) 59, 77, 78, 99
Heart attack 57, 58, 79, 116, 117
Heart disease 172, 238
Heart failure 116, 117
Helping hand 228
Hiding medicines 164
HIV 117, 118
Hoist 48
Home adaptations 51
Hot water bottle 62
Household hazards 39
Household tasks 218-223
Human body 70-93
Human immunodeficiency virus (HIV) 117, 118
Hydration 129, 151
Hypertonia 112
Hypo 65
Hypoglycaemia 65
Hypothermia 118
Hypotonia 112

Telephone receiver stand 232
Terminal care 148-154
Thermostatic mixing valve 200
Thrombosis 79
Time-sheets 21
Tinnitus 89
Toilet, using the 205-206, 208-216
Toenails 74, 203
Tongue 92, 169
Toothpaste dispenser 231
Toilet seats 231
Toothbrush handles 231
Trachea 78
Transfer sling 229
Transport 44, 169, 190
Tray 228, 229, 232
Tremor 119
Trip hazards 39
Trolley 229
Tumours 82, 92, 112, 115, 132
Tunnel vision 85, 86
Turban 191

U

UKHCA (United Kingdom Homecare Association) 1, 3, 8, 25
Unconscious 57, 64, 66, 112, 118
Unsafe equipment 47
Unsaturated fat 172
Urge incontinence 210
Urinary incontinence 208, 210-211, 212
Urinary infection 28, 109, 211
Urinary system 79
Urine 79, 81, 92, 109, 170, 206, 208, 210, 211, 214, 215, 216, 230

Urine bottle 214, 230
User satisfaction survey 25

V

Vagina 80
Vascular dementia 114, 122
Vegetables 42, 170, 171, 173, 177, 178, 182
Violent behaviour 34, 66, 67, 123, 127, 128
Vitamins 168, 171, 173
Vitamin B1 deficiency 132
Vocational qualification 6, 24
Vomiting 42, 169

W

Walking 110
Walking aids 73, 240
Walking frame 73
Walking stick 72, 229
Washing
 - *clothes* 81
 - *eyes* 84
 - *food* 42, 178, 182
 - *hands (careworkers)* 40, 41, 109, 178, 182, 199
 - *kitchen utensils* 42, 179, 182
 - *service users* 74, 81, 125, 146, 198, 200-201, 205, 215, 229
 - *service users - checklist* 205-06
 - *service users in bed* 204
 - *wheelchair cushions* 215
Washing Machine 41